BEHIND THE SMILE

A story of life after loss

MITCH McPHERSON

BEHIND THE SMILE:
A story of life after loss

ISBN 9780648218081

Published by

Mitch McPherson
www.mitchmcpherson.com.au

First published 2018

Designed by Julie Hawkins, In Graphic Detail
Printed in Australia by Griffin Press
Set in 10 pt on 13 pt Adagio

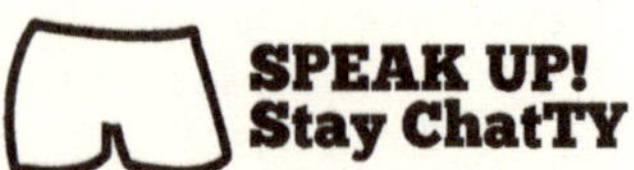

A portion of the proceeds from sales of this book will be donated to **SPEAK UP! Stay ChatTY**

"Behind the Smile takes us to a place that nobody ever wants to go and opens our eyes to the profound impact of suicide. Mitch McPherson shares his deeply personal story about the day that everything changed, how he has found true purpose and how we can all look a bit deeper at those around us who might be struggling.

Mitch, this can't have been an easy story to write so thanks for sharing it with such honesty and sensitivity. Time spent reading this will be time well spent for anyone.

Your passion and commitment always inspires me Mitch and is a testament to the love and respect you have for your brother Ty and everyone who loves and misses him."

—Brendan Maher
CEO, R U OK?

"Mitch, I'm so proud of what you, your family and everyone is doing with this book and SPEAK UP! Stay ChatTY. It takes a lot of courage to constantly relive a devastating situation for the education of others.

Sharing your experience in what you noticed in Ty over his last month is the legacy you and this book will leave forever — your legacy is a true lifesaver. Your actions are of a person who looks outside of themselves for the benefit of people you may or may not know.

Somewhere Ty is still watching you and still copying your every move and action. No doubt he's grinning from ear to ear, proud to have you as his older brother."

—Jack Riewoldt
AFL footballer

ACKNOWLEDGEMENTS

Ty McPherson
Sahar McPherson
Dale and Koula McPherson-Taylor
Vicki and Glenn Stevens
Nan Norma and Pop John
Grandma Maxine
Jenna McPherson
Brock and Ruby Voss
Emmanuel Tsakiris
Athina Tsakiris
Michaela Delmadoros
Maritza Atzamoglue
Saad Mohamad
Najla Mohamad
Hassan Mohamad
Sleiman Mohamad
Haidar Mohamad

Hilary Burden (co-writer)
Clive Tilsley (support)
Julie Hawkins (designer)
Julia Gandy (support editor)

Stay ChatTY/ Relationships Australia Tasmania team members (Mat Rowell, Michael Kelly, Amanda French, Julia Gandy, James Rice, Kat Pullen, Jane Garvey)
Stay ChatTY committee members (Paul Lyons, Dan Morgan, Brad Dutton, Hayley Dodge, Brett Garth, Tom McMeekin)

Friends and extended family, you all know who you are.

Brendan Maher
Jack Riewoldt

DJ Motors
Banjos
Zest
St Lukes
NAB

To all that have helped make SPEAK UP! Stay ChatTY what it is today.

Lastly, to all who are reading this book, thank YOU!!

CONTENTS

For Ty, and for every person who has lost someone to suicide

This story was inspired by my little brother Ty, who took his own life ten days after his 18th birthday. It contains descriptions of my experience of his suicide death and its aftermath.

If reading this book causes you distress or you feel you need support, please call Lifeline on 13 11 14 or visit www.staychatty.com.au/get-help/ for more information.

CHAPTER 1

January 14, 2013

THIS ISN'T REAL, this can't be real, this is not real ... The same words are coming back to me, over and over again. It's as if my brain is stuck in one gear. Tears stream down my face. I try to wipe them away with the sleeve of a hoodie — one my mate Duck lent me to stop me shivering — but they just keep coming. My mouth is dry as dirt. I want to vomit, swallowing instead, doing my best to hold everything inside. I feel weak, numb all over, slumped over the arm of Mum's couch. It's dark outside. The lounge room blinds are closed. All I can hear are the desperate sounds of people sobbing uncontrollably.

It's late on Monday night. Dad has had to coax me up the front path to Mum's house. I'd normally be at his place, a seven-minute drive away, brushing my teeth and getting ready for bed.

"I don't want to go inside. I don't want to see it," I say to Dad through tears.

I can see he is a mess, too. I feel an arm around my neck, pulling me in for a big hug.

"I understand," he says, "but think about it mate. Just make sure you won't regret it in years to come."

My immediate family has gathered together outside. Dad, my step-mum Koula, Mum, my step-dad Glenn, sister Jenna, step-brother Emmanuel, Nan and

Pop, and Grandma Maxine. I can taste and smell the fear that seems to drench us as, one by one, we slowly make our way inside the house. Up the stairs, through the open front door, into the hallway.

We know what we're about to walk in to do, but none of us is ready. To this day I'm not sure where we found the strength – but we did.

My girlfriend, Sahar, is urging me to go inside while she waits with the rest of our friends and extended family gathered across the front yard. No one is speaking. There are just tears. I am the last to go in and I walk inside.

Usually, it's an everyday, unremarkable kind of walk to Mum's house. I'd pop in once a week to see her and Glenn. I was always a "too busy for Mum" kinda guy. I'd just want to say a quick hello, answer all her questions about what was happening in my life, talk footy with Glenn, and be on my way.

Tonight is different.

Three paramedics and two police officers are standing at the entrance to the hallway. I can see in their eyes the hurt and sadness they feel for us. Dad is having a quiet word with one of the paramedics. He puts an arm round Dad's shoulder and says, "Take your time mate".

I am waiting in the hallway for my turn to enter the lounge room. I've heard every scream, every sob. My breathing speeds up, my heart is beating out of my chest. On top of everything, Nan has had to be taken to hospital. She had existing heart trouble and, being emotional and upset, we had to call a second ambulance for her.

"Pop, how is this happening?" I say. None of it feels real.

It's my turn. Slowly I go through the door. The lights are off. The lounge is filled with the soft, flickering light of Mums' candles, lit by family and friends and placed around the room. In the middle, on a metal ambulance trolley, with a white sheet up to his face, is my young brother Ty.

Just a few hours earlier, Ty had come home from spending the morning with Dad, gone into his bedroom and killed himself.

We gather around Ty's body. Most of us are holding on to someone or the nearest piece of furniture for support, as if we've lost every bone in our body. Jenna is inconsolable and can't let go of her dead brother. She is on his right side lying across him with her head on his stomach. Mum is at his feet, screaming and wailing, "Oh Ty, why my boy?" Glenn is also beside himself. Ty was the son that Glenn never had. And it was Glenn who had found Ty that afternoon.

Dad is on his knees with Ty's hand in his. His head is pressed up against Ty's and he is speaking into his ear, telling him to wake up, and how much he loves him.

I am watching from afar feeling nothing but numbness, still thinking this cannot be happening. After a few minutes – I have no idea how long, time seems irrelevant – I move towards Ty, shaking and scared. Dad steps back a bit to allow me to get closer. I place the back of my right hand on his face. He still feels warm. I'll never forget the shade of blue in and around his face. I'd never seen a lifeless body before, only in movies. I just couldn't believe this was my little brother's.

I lean in and put my head on Ty's chest, mumbling and sobbing for my little brother to wake up. Someone grabs me, holding me tight from behind as I become inconsolable trying to hug Ty. "No, no, no," I continue to say, holding his lifeless body in my arms.

Sahar has been sitting on the lawn of the neighbour's house up from Mum's. She watches alone in tears as everyone turns up, their cars pulling up on either side of the street. My mate Timmy has spotted her and sits down beside her. Neither of them can believe what is happening and don't know what to do.

Eventually I come out of the house to get Sahar. We'd only been going out for a short while, and she hadn't even met Mum yet. I lead Sahar on to the front balcony and introduce them.

"I'm so sorry we have to meet on such horrible circumstances," Sahar says.

Mum is in an absolute state, but still she gives Sahar a hug.

Later, outside, standing in between Sahar and Timmy, we watch as Ty's body, wrapped in a sheet, is carried downstairs on the trolley and loaded into the back of a hearse. The paramedics are taking Ty for a post-mortem. We watch as the sombre vehicle drives down the road and out of sight. Timmy says we'd been in the lounge room with Ty for more than 20 minutes. Everything is a blur.

I do my best not to think about that evening. When I do look back, I have sleepless nights remembering how I watched my family go into the house to see Ty for the very last time. Sahar remembers Pop completely and utterly shocked, saying over and over in his distinctive Greek accent, "Why, why is this happening?"

That night had been a real-life nightmare – one none of us saw coming.

It was also the night that our family had officially been welcomed into the dark, terrifying, and brutal world of suicide.

CHAPTER 2

Growing up

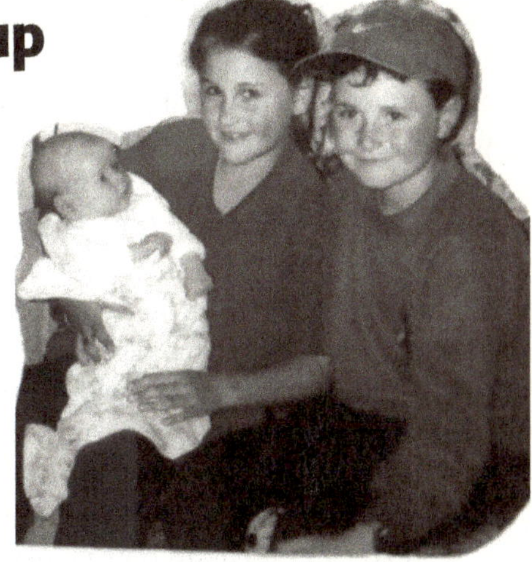

My sister Jenna here at age 6 holding Ty. I was 8 at the time and we were both very proud and excited to have a new younger brother.

I WAS THE FIRST of three children, born on August 28, 1987 in Hobart, Tasmania. My Mum, Vicki, is one of three daughters born to parents Con and Norma. Mum's sisters, Maritza and Eleni, have eight children between them. Dad had one brother, sons to Kevin and Maxine, and a stepsister, Mandy. My parents had my sister Jenna in 1989, and Ty was born six years later in 1995.

We grew up on Hobart's eastern shore and moved house quite a bit. Dad was a butcher until he began working at the prison as a custodial officer in 2006. Mum looked after the three kids while working part-time jobs along the way. Before Dad started working at the prison we didn't have a lot of money as a family. At times we knew money was tight, but my parents worked hard to provide for us, and were able to send us to private schools.

We had a great childhood. There was always something going on — barbecues, family visits, and weekends away. But we were far from perfect.

Mum and Dad separated when I was 13. They hadn't been happy for quite a while and I remember feeling a sense of relief when Dad finally packed up and moved into his own place. It had been brewing for a while until it finally happened. One Saturday we were in the car, when an argument broke out and got so bad that Mum pulled over and Dad got out. I jumped out with him, while Mum drove off with Jenna and Ty still in the backseat. I will never forget watching our beat-up white station wagon speed off up the road.

Dad and I have always had a strong father-son relationship. I didn't choose him over Mum that day, but I felt I needed to get out with him. I remember leaning on a rusty fence by the side of the road, crying.

"I just can't do it anymore with your Mum," Dad said. "We just aren't meant to be".

It was the first heartfelt conversation Dad and I had ever had.

Sometimes I sit and think about life and what it would have been like if they hadn't separated and remained a happy, loving couple. Separations are tumultuous. They hit people hard. It is tough to watch your parents fight and scream and argue. I know Jenna and I were old enough to understand what was going on. But Ty, who was 10 at the time, may not have been able to grasp it so easily. I wonder what effect their separation had on him. Nowadays, parents seem to separate all the time. But back then, for a young boy in primary school, it must have been a lot to deal with. He was always staying between houses, and never really settled into his own permanent bedroom until he was a teenager.

When Mum and Dad broke up, in the beginning we stayed mostly with Mum, but after a while I went to live with Dad. I stayed with Dad until I moved into my own home in 2016.

The best house Dad and I lived in was in just outside Hobart. I was working full time as a glazier and Dad was doing shift work at the prison, so I had plenty of time on my own at home while Dad was at work. My mates were always visiting, playing backyard cricket, having Saturday beer sessions, or hungover Sunday sessions by the wood fire.

My relationship with Ty was always strong, but it wasn't until life between Mum and Dad had finally settled down that he and I got closer. Ty spent most of his time with Mum after the separation, but as things settled, he started staying more with me at Dad's.

Jenna and Ty were extremely close. When he was very young Jenna's nickname for him was 'Tig' and it stuck for the rest of his life. Jenna has two children, and when they were young, Ty was an amazing uncle to them. He played with them, baby-sat, showered them with gifts, but most of all he cared for and loved them.

My Nanny Norma was the absolute light of so many worlds, short in stature, but larger than life. Nan was one of those people who just said what she wanted

My Nanny Norma loved the camera and was always happy to pose for a photo.

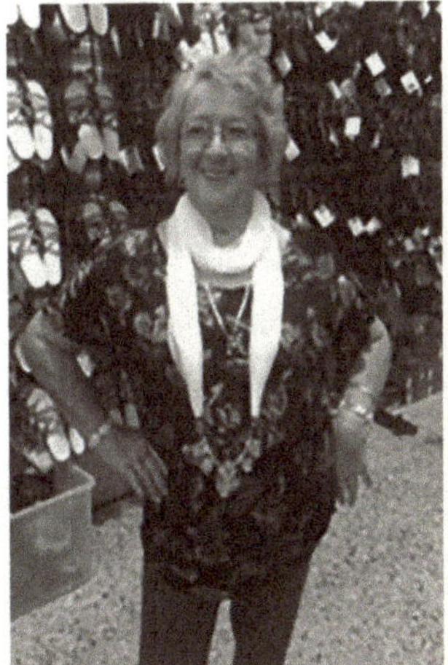

Ty displaying love to his new nephew Brock summed up his passion for being a loving uncle.

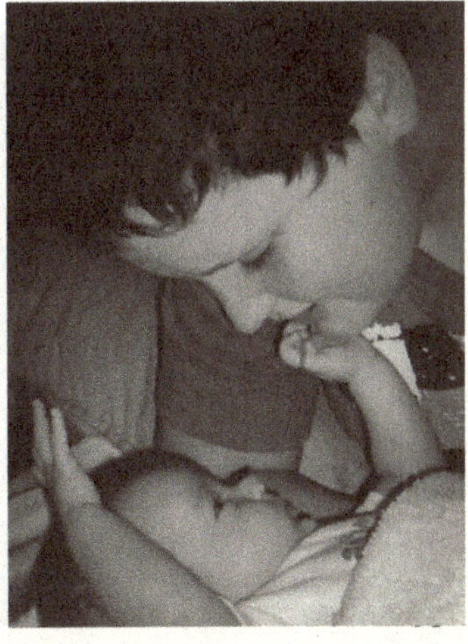

without worrying what people thought. Normally I wouldn't consider this trait a virtue, but Nan was inappropriate in a good way. If she thought one of her family members was putting on weight, she would tell them – in front of everyone! She would ask crude questions and didn't mind telling a dirty joke, especially after a wine or two.

Nan and Pop had over 15 grandchildren and great-grandchildren. Among them were Ty, Ry and Eli, which confused the life out of Nan. It was the funniest thing when Nan couldn't get out the right name when talking about one of the grandkids. Sometimes it took five or six trys.

Pop was the handy man who loved to spend time by himself – fishing, under the house or in his beloved hothouse. Quite often, I'd see Pop's car parked outside a local betting agency. He loved to call in and dabble on the horses to pass the time. Renowned for his cooked fish in the pan, Pop simply loved providing for his family and enjoyed having happy people around him.

Ty in the middle with my sister Jenna and me. Ty's freckles starting to sprout just like his big brother.

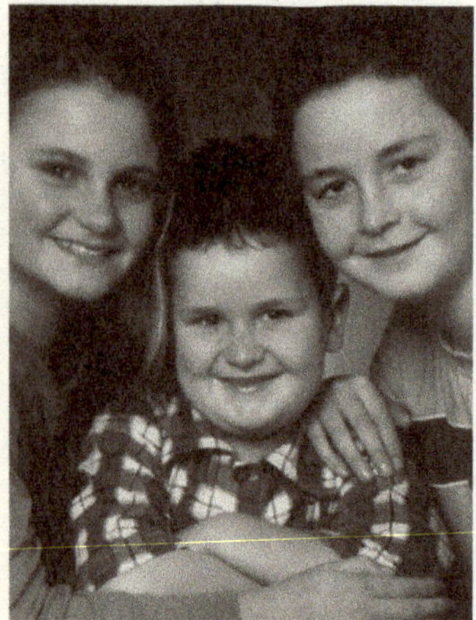

Unlike Nan, Pop wasn't a huge fan of a photo. But he certainly did love being around his family and taking care of the ones he loved.

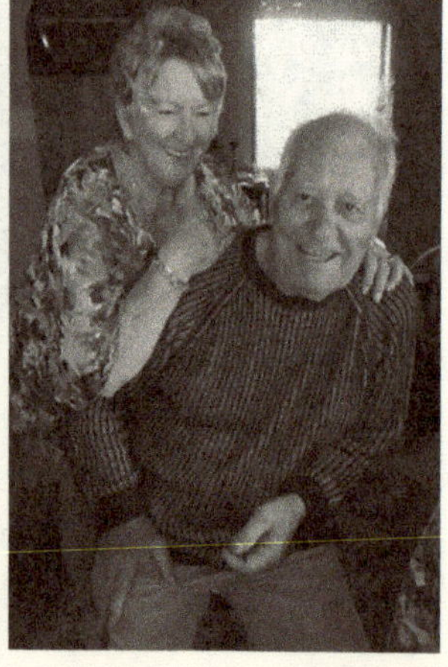

I cared so much for my little brother, and I am proud to say that I was his idol. Growing up he always wanted to be around me, talk like me, do the things I did. He even wanted to dress like me. We wrestled, we played backyard cricket, we kicked the footy – all the normal things that those lucky enough to grow up with a brother get to do.

There were so many times when I would groan and whinge about receiving one of his, "Hey, where are you?" texts – which usually meant, "Can you come and pick me up?". But I always did it. Every chance I had I would flick him some money to buy lunch. It made me feel better to know he had money on him. I still cry whenever I think about his cheery little face lighting up, showering me with gratitude when I slipped him a $10 note.

AS A TEENAGER I worked at Woolworths. I enjoyed working there and met a lot of people I still see out and about today. I worked hard, but I didn't exactly have my priorities in order at the time. It was approaching AFL Grand Final day in 2005, and unfortunately for me, my manager had rostered me on to work that Saturday. I did everything I could to get out of it. I even organised someone to fill my shift. To my dismay, my manager wouldn't let me change it, so I did what I shouldn't have, and I resigned.

Four months later, I finished my second year of college. I wanted to get an apprenticeship but had no idea in which trade. I was open to taking anything I could get by this stage. One Saturday, I was flicking through the jobs section of the paper and spotted a glazing apprenticeship with a business north of Hobart. I applied the following Monday, and, after a week, much to my relief, I got the job.

My employer, Scott, was a local cricketer who had set up his own business from scratch and was finally making the move to take on new staff. I completed a four-year apprenticeship and worked for Scott for over seven years. We had a great relationship and he was a big influence on my professional skills and work ethic.

Glaziers spend a lot of time on the tools, but Scott prided us on customer service and good communication. A big part of my role was engaging with customers, and I found that I was actually really good at it. I also enjoyed it – a bonus. Eventually I ran the business and managed staff when Scott and his wife took holidays. We were a small business in a saturated market of small glazing businesses, so I knew it was important to show good work ethic with customers: cleanliness, organisation, and a good finished product. But I could never have known how learning to communicate well and lead others to achieve results would put me in such good stead for the not-for-profit I would go on to found seven years later. It was as if I was being prepared for a future that was still unknown to me.

I enjoyed glazing, but I wasn't passionate about it. I loved the boys I worked with, we had some fun days on the tools, and I liked wearing tradie shorts and Blunnies every day. My work was rarely in one spot, always going from job to job which I liked, being quite an impatient person. My next step would have been to start my own business. I kept putting off, telling myself that one day I'd make the leap. But I never found the drive to do it.

For seven and a half years I worked an 8am to 4pm day. Then it was off to the gym or footy training – or both. I played in the Tasmanian State League until the age of 23. After that, the commitment got a bit much so a few of us decided to drop a league to play in the Old Scholars League. It was the best decision we could have made. After three years of being a bottom-tier team, we finally won the Premiership in 2011. We didn't lose a game all season and went through 20-0. To cap off a good year, I was lucky enough to win 'Best On Ground' in the Grand Final.

That day is one of my fondest sporting memories. Every time I think of it I remember the smile on the faces of two people I loved so much: my Dad, and my Nan Norma. I have plenty of photos from that day and one with Nan I especially love. She didn't know anything about footy, and could never have realised how awesome it was for me to have won a flag and 'Best On'. But I remember her saying, "Oh my boy, I am so proud of you", right before we had our photograph taken at the oval.

In the time before Ty died, my girlfriend Sahar and I had been together for less than a year, and I was looking forward to a future with her – going on holidays, spending time with her family, and of doing something with my life that would inspire me.

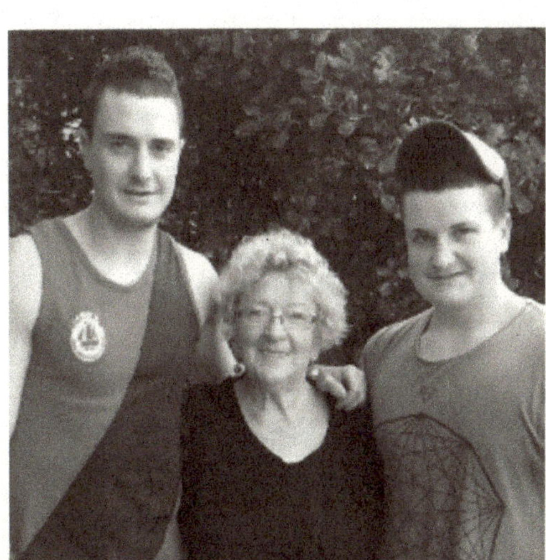

I used to finish football training and call into Mum's on my way home to say hello. I always loved it when Nan was there, and on this occasion, a rare photo of me with Nan and Ty.

Sahar is the best thing that has ever happened to me. She is loyal, hardworking, driven, and drop dead gorgeous (I have been told a thousand times I am batting above my average). She is more supportive than anyone I know. Meeting her and being welcomed into her family brought and still brings me more joy than I can imagine. And Sahar loved Ty. She loved his kindness and his cheeky smile. He loved her sense of humour, and how she bagged me out in front of him.

But it wasn't all smooth sailing. Sahar is Muslim, and it wasn't in Sahar's parents' minds that she would ever meet and fall in love with an Australian, especially a light-skinned Australian boy. Arabs tend to marry Arabs, and Sahar's family expected the same of her. It's important for them to maintain the strong cultural and religious traditions they are raised with, so Sahar worried I would not be accepted.

We weren't exactly honest to Sahar's parents about being together. In fact, they had no idea. For a year and a half we managed to keep it from them, a tricky time to say the least. I would constantly ask "When can I meet the family?" But Sahar wanted to

I don't think I ever knew the true meaning of a "selfie" until I met my beautiful wife Sahar. Weekends away with her are what I treasure — here we are at Tasmania's Cradle Mountain.

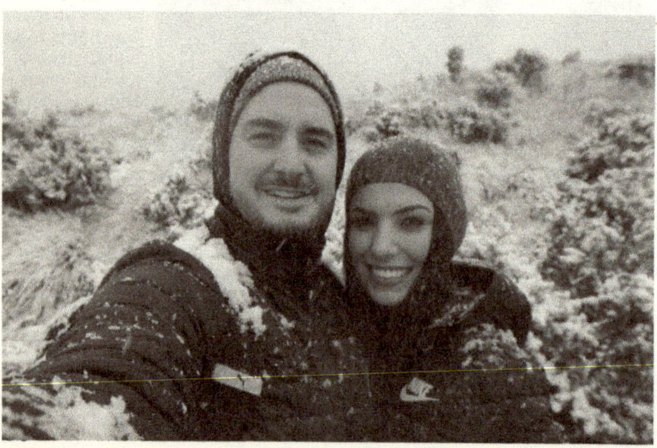

be absolutely certain that I was the one before taking that step. It was hard to understand that at the time, but looking back now I respect the way she did it. It took a lot of courage and faith in me for her to tell her parents, "I've met a boy. Oh, and he's an Aussie".

Telstra 4G
3:28 pm
54%
Sahar ▸ Mitch McPherson
14 January 2013 · Bellerive, TAS
I'll forever be here for you!
Love you <3
Like
Comment
Maritza and 9 others
Mitch McPherson
I love you xx
5y Like
2

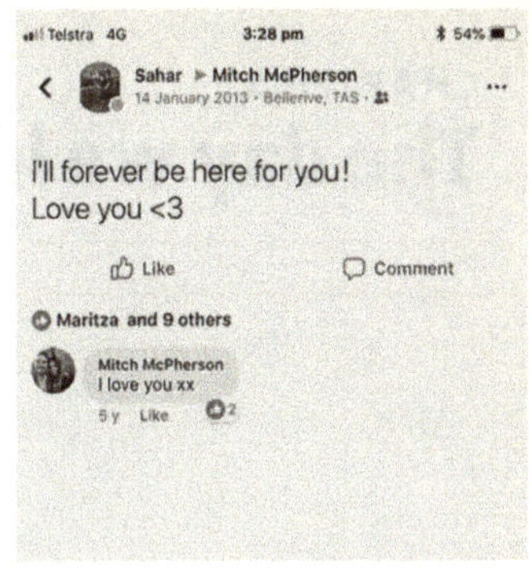

I will never forget this first public show of commitment from Sahar. Just what I needed in my time of absolute despair.

The night we lost Ty, I remember looking at Sahar, watching her crying and thinking to myself, "She is going to have to tell her parents what has happened". I asked her what she was going to say. There was no way she could go home and act like nothing was wrong – she was a mess.

Because of our situation we had rarely been outwardly affectionate, or made it obvious we were together – much to my disappointment. But that night, she told me she loved me. It was the first time she had said it. I remember her message popping up on my phone, and in the midst of that darkest tornado, I felt a flicker of light go off in my heart. She knew how much that would mean to me.

BEFORE WE LOST TY, we weren't the perfect family and I certainly wasn't the perfect son or brother. I loved the people around me, but went through life with blinders on, ignorant to the problems others faced and focusing on myself. I certainly didn't understand anything about mental ill-health or suicide, and never thought they would have anything to do with me or my family.

CHAPTER 3
The day we lost Ty

MONDAY morning, my first day back at work after nearly four weeks off over Christmas. I had been absolutely dreading it for days. It's a shock to the system, returning to work after holidays. I loved the people I worked with – my boss, his family, and the boys got me through most days – but that didn't lessen the dread of going back to something I didn't love.

My alarm went off 6:40am. Already you could tell it was going to be a warm Hobart day.

After snoozing my alarm four or five times I finally got up, had a shower, and put on my tradie gear. I gathered my things for work, had a quick chat to Dad before heading off. Koula ran a local take away so Dad was always up early to see her off.

Dad hit the kettle to make another cup of tea, and took it outside to potter about the backyard.

"What time are you heading out?" I yelled to Dad through the screen door.

The night before Dad mentioned that he and Ty were going shopping to get some new work boots and tradie shorts. Ty was starting an apprenticeship in Hobart the next day. Then they were going to visit his new boss and work mates to check in and get to know them.

"Ah, about mid-morning I reckon. We'll go and have some brekkie as soon as Tig gets out of bed."

"OK, nice" I replied. "Have a good one. I'll see you tonight." I shut the screen door and headed back through the house and out to my car, and set off on my 40-minute drive to work.

I got to work and said hello to my colleagues. We laughed and spoke about holidays. We were all a bit slow and lacked motivation given it was day one of the new year.

The boss arrived to allocate our work for the day, and to my excitement, he only gave me two job sheets for the whole day. It was like Christmas all over again, bound to be a cruisy day to ease back into work. I drove out of the shed thinking what an idiot I'd been, ruining the last few days of my holidays dreading going back to work, when it couldn't have been easier.

Back to reality, back into the working world. I bowled my first job over by about 10am, and the second major job by 1pm. Other things came in, but the day managed to pass slowly, without feeling that I had been run off my feet. I spent a lot of time on my phone – Facebook, Instagram, WhatsApp with the boys, texting Sahar and my friends.

But there's one text I will never forget. I still have it in my phone, received from Ty that morning at 10:04am.

Hey, do you still have one of those fourfold rulers for work?

I replied about an hour and a half later, at 11:33am.

I'll get back to you in a tick. I'll look in my toolbox.

I looked inside my toolbox at least a dozen times that day. And each time, the bright yellow fourfold ruler was staring me right in the face. But I didn't message him.

At 4:30pm, I finally finished work for the day.

"Catch you later, I'm heading home," I yelled to the boys.

When I jumped in my ute I realised I still hadn't replied to Ty's text. All day I had been on my phone, yet I went the whole day without getting back to Ty to let him know that I had the ruler he was looking for, and that I'd get it to him at home that night. How could I have been so complacent? I headed out of the driveway, pulled over to the side of the road, and got my phone out to call Ty and have a chat.

Ty's name is still third on my list of favourites in my phone, under my two best mates Timmy and Ben. He didn't answer, but that didn't surprise me or raise any alarm bells. It wasn't unusual for Ty not to answer his phone. He was a bit of a ratbag with it, and it would drive us all crazy. Sometimes he'd call, I'd miss it, I'd call straight back and he wouldn't answer. I used to ask him, "Do you call people, and when they don't answer, just throw your phone away?"

I knew I'd catch him as soon as I got home, so I put the phone down and set off again.

It was 5:10pm by the time I got home to Dad's. Dad and Koula were in the kitchen as I snacked on some food and asked about their day. I had a shower and put on some shorts and a singlet. It was a stinking hot afternoon. Dad was still there when I made my way back upstairs to the kitchen for a glass of water.

"Have you heard from Ty?" Dad asked. "I dropped him at your Mum's about 1:30pm after we'd been out and about. He said he was going to pack a bag, then come straight down and spend the night with us."

"No, I haven't," I told Dad. "He texted me earlier and I tried to call him but he didn't answer. I'm sure he'll be here soon."

About an hour and a half passed, and it was nearing 7pm. Sahar finally arrived which meant it was dinnertime.

We were downstairs in my bedroom having a conversation – actually, more of a silly argument – about what we were going to eat for dinner. Sahar now knows the full story and I have since been busted for lying. I told her I had been given a huge workload and that I was too tired to go upstairs and cook for her like I'd promised. Sahar sat on my bed with her back up against the steel bedhead. I stood at the foot as we argued, until my phone started to ring in my pocket.

I pulled it out, looked at it, and saw it was Mum calling. Back then, she was notorious for checking in on us three kids every couple of days, ringing with the usual Mum questions: "What have you been doing?" "What have you been eating?" or "When are you coming to see me?"

I rolled my eyes and thought, "I can't be bothered answering that right now". I was hungry and keen to get some food.

"I'll give her a call back later," I said to Sahar, throwing the phone on my bed.

A few seconds later, right up above us, we heard Dad let out an enormous cry. Then Koula screamed, louder than Dad.

I stared at Sahar on the bed.

"What the fuck?" I cried out.

Both of us were frozen, too afraid to move, wondering what the bloody hell was going on upstairs. The next ten seconds felt like an eternity, as we heard them both running around, yelling and screaming.

It was pure pandemonium.

Eventually I realised I'd better head upstairs and find out what was happening. I opened the door, started running up the stairs, and reached half way when I saw Dad flying out of the kitchen with a look on his face I will never forget: the look of utter fear. It was clear that something terrible had happened.

"Ty has killed himself," Dad screamed, breathless and panicked. "We are going up to your mother's".

I caught my breath and screamed, "What the fuck?" again. "What? What? How?"

"Your mother rang. Ambulance is there now".

Up at Mum's place, Mum's husband Glenn had arrived home from work a bit after 6pm. He knew Mum wouldn't be home until late and didn't think Ty was home either, so he went outside to water the lawn. After a while Glenn came back inside. He spotted Ty's thongs in the hallway, along with a note that had been placed on the table by the front door.

"Hey Tig!" he called out. "How are you going?"

No one answered, so he went to Ty's bedroom. The door was shut. He tried to open it, but it seemed stuck. He forced his way in to find Ty's lifeless body.

"GO!" I yelled.

Dad and Koula jumped into their green Pajero and flew off up the road.

I raced back downstairs. Sahar had heard Dad tell me the news.

All I felt was disbelief, and a steadily rising panic.

"No. No. No. No," I kept saying, pacing around the room.

I was deathly pale as Sahar took control and said, "We have to get up there".

My first reaction wasn't to go. I was so scared, I didn't know what to feel or think. I got my phone out to ring Mum back – I needed to hear it for myself – but she didn't answer.

"Let's go then," I said, and we both ran out of my room and up the stairs. We jumped into Sahar's car, and like Dad, took off at a pace up the street.

The trip was the longest drive of my life – no more than ten minutes, but it felt like hours. I rocked backwards and forwards, yelling at Sahar to drive faster, but she was going as fast as she could. Sahar was petrified, doing her best to stay calm while I just couldn't take in what was happening.

As we neared the street, Sahar pulled over to let me out. We could see directly up to Mum's place. So much was happening: ambulances were parked across the lawn and driveway, lights flashing, neighbours were gathering around. I could hear crying and screaming, even from outside.

I told Sahar I wanted to go up to the house alone. She hadn't met Mum yet, and I just couldn't deal with them meeting amidst this chaos.

It was real. This nightmare was actually happening to us, and there was nothing I could do.

I got out of the car, bare foot, and sprinted up to the house. I was crying, and kept saying "no" under my breath, cursing Ty, thinking he better not have done this. I got halfway when Dad came out of the open front door. His hands were on his head. I fell in a heap on the footpath, sobbing, struggling with a kind of pain I had never felt before. I was all but crawling on the ground, screaming, crying out for Ty.

I couldn't breathe and couldn't get up until Sahar knelt down behind me. The news had hit her too because she was a mess. "Come on, come on," she repeated, almost picking me up and dragging me toward Mum's house.

When we finally made it to the front lawn, I saw Mum was on the deck. I still didn't know if Ty was alive or not. Something was stopping me going up the steps and going inside. I didn't want it confirmed. To become real.

"I just can't do it," I told Sahar desperately. "I don't want to go in there."

I shouted out to Mum, who was leaning at the front door. "What is going on?"

She couldn't speak properly, but finally mumbled back, "They're still working on Ty, they're all in there."

When Jenna arrived, she was a mess. She went straight to Ty's bedroom but was held back by a police officer who told her she couldn't go in.

It was chaos. So much of that night is a blur. At one stage, Koula ran down the stairs, speaking on the phone to her son.

"Emmanuel, Ty's dead. He's killed himself," she cried out.

"Shut the fuck up," I shouted. "Don't shout it out like that! Don't yell it out!"

I wish I hadn't spoken to Koula that way. But what was going on was so raw, so unimaginable, I just couldn't understand it, let alone have it said out loud like that. I couldn't accept that it was true.

Twenty minutes later, the paramedics came outside and declared Ty deceased.

Dad came out of Ty's bedroom onto the front deck, his face blank and his eyes hollow.

"Are you going to come in?" he asked quietly.

"Is he dead?" I asked.

I heard someone say yes.

Mum was on the deck. Other people had started to arrive and were gathered around the front door. Finally, I went up the steps and hugged Mum. She was beside herself. People were crying, sobbing, staring into the distance, wondering how the hell this had happened.

A paramedic eventually came out and spoke to us. He told us that Ty had gone, and that they were preparing him so we could see him.

More and more people started to arrive. Neighbours were standing in their driveways wondering what was going on with all the police cars and ambulances at Mum's. Ty's friends were there, Jenna's friends, all my mates, family friends. They circled around, heads down, not knowing what to do. I was freezing cold, so my mate Duck leant me his hoodie. When Sahar and I had raced out of the house earlier we hadn't thought to grab anything. I still wasn't wearing any shoes.

It was close to midnight by the time people started to leave. It was extremely hard to have to leave, but I managed to say goodnight to Mum and her family. We left to go back home to Dad's place. Koula drove, my grandmother, Maxine, next to her in the front seat, and I sat in the back with Dad. I felt his arm around me all the way home.

The last thought I had was of the letter on the hall table. Ty had left a handwritten note – the one Glenn had found when he'd come inside. Ty's words were churning in my mind on the short drive home. On one side, it said:

I love each and every one of you so much ...

And on the other:

I'm sorry – Love always.

CHAPTER 4

My brother Ty

TY WAS BORN on January 4, 1995 in Hobart. He had dark, curly hair, brown eyes, and chubby features. People used to call him a "Mini Mitch".

He was a quiet boy growing up, but smiled at everyone he met. Although he didn't play a lot of organised team sports, he enjoyed getting stuck into sports at home or on the weekends, and as a devoted Carlton supporter, loved watching his footy on TV. He was a larrikin among his friends, and loved getting a laugh and creating some fun. But mostly he was a shy, caring guy who only knew how to be kind to those around him.

I know parents aren't supposed to have favourites but I think Ty was Mum and Dad's. They both had an amazing relationship with him. He was their baby. Jenna and I were grown up. We were hanging out with friends and playing sport, while Ty was still happy to go visiting friends with Mum, or spend time under the house tinkering away with Dad.

One of the funniest things about Ty growing up was his difficulty saying words containing the letter "s". He always replaced the "s" with "f"! My sister and I found endless entertainment in asking Ty to say words like "suck". One of my good mate's nicknames was "Swanny". I still call him "Fwanny".

Before high school, Ty had been reserved in public. He had lacked a little in self-confidence through his early teens after he'd been hit in the eye with a dart. He was only 12 when he had surgery to fix it. Unable to move or exercise for a long time, he gained weight and that challenged him at that stage. At home though, he was always the life of the party: laughing, making fun of all of us, revelling in conversation. He lit up our home life.

Ty enjoyed most sports growing up, but didn't really start playing footy again until high school. I was delighted to see my little brother was into sports – and through it, building a great group of friends. I used to see him and his mates at the local footy, or at the Big Bash cricket, and they were just like my mates and me. They were starting to dress the same as us, talk like us, even have the same sense of humour as us. I was always reassured knowing he was a popular young kid.

Aside from the eye injury, starting around age 15, Ty complained about having a bad back. This persisted until his death. There were days when he could only lie in bed, upset and in pain. Dad had taken him to the doctor and the physiotherapist a few times, but it never seemed to get better. I had a few conversations with him about his back, but didn't take the time to really understand what he was going through. Instead, I was dealing with my own life issues – petty in comparison – and putting myself first. I never really knuckled down to find out why he had a bad back, even though I knew firsthand how back pain makes you irritable. I never reached out to help him deal with it.

I feel that guilt. It upsets me that I didn't try to help Ty. We don't know if physical pain contributed to his death, but we do know mental health can be impacted by physical pain.

For Sahar, my younger brother was a "mini Mitch," with the biggest smile. Her fondest memory of Ty was when he came to tell us his neighbour, an elderly man, had given him all the shirts he no longer wore. Ty, being the kind soul that he was, accepted them with a big smile on his face, and came in to show us all these shirts. He was never going to wear them but didn't want to break the old man's heart. Sahar wondered what 17-year-old boy would do that. She always thought of him as a beautiful boy.

Ty was the last person you would think was going through a difficult time. The family and friends who knew him saw him as someone cheery, engaged and gaining confidence. He was tall, shedding his baby fat, and turning into a handsome young man, just like his brother.

IN THE FIRST WEEK of 2013, we had just celebrated Ty's 18th birthday. We had dinner at a pub in the city, and continued on for drinks at a couple of nightclubs. I saw Ty drinking and dancing that Saturday night, and it was an absolute blowout. Finally seeing Ty with his friends was really fun, but odd to reconcile with the Ty I knew. My baby brother all grown up. I remember telling him we hadn't done that before, drinking and partying together. Later we joked about sharing our first hangover.

Opposite, clockwise from top left: My favourite picture of Ty as a toddler.

A rare photo of Ty and me together at Mum's house, chatting on the couch.

Ty was always excited to see Dad when he got home from work after a shift.

This picture shows Ty's shy side: that was how many knew him.

One of my favourite photos of Mum and Ty.

The three of us heading out for a Father's day dinner with Dad in 2010. This photo will forever remain my Facebook cover photo.

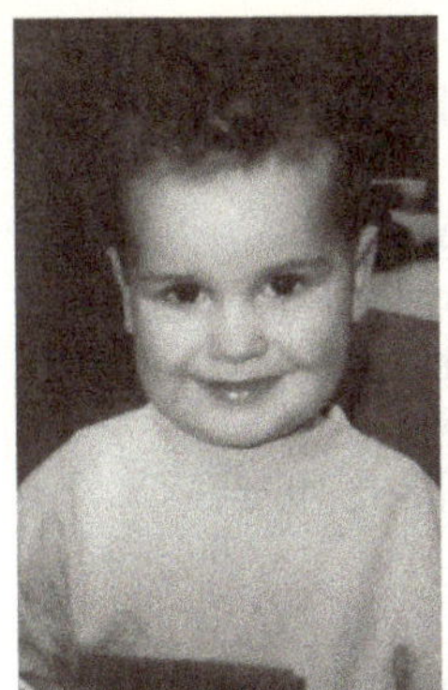

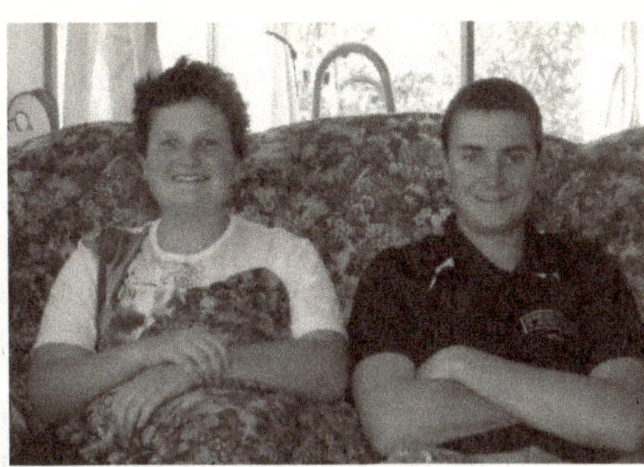

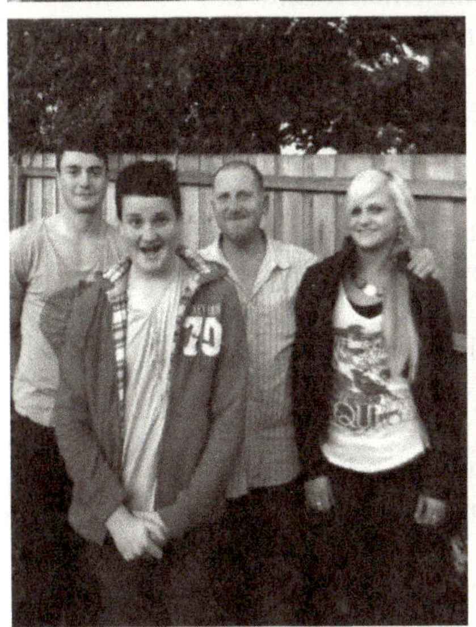

70

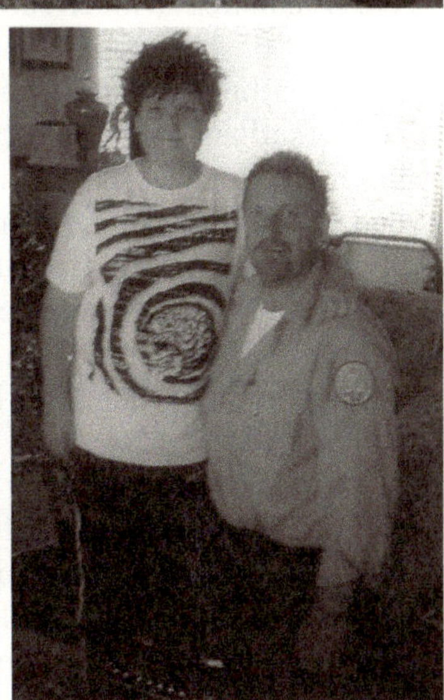

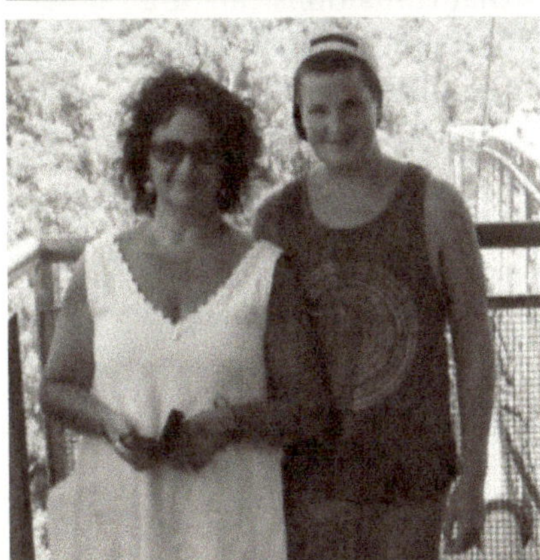

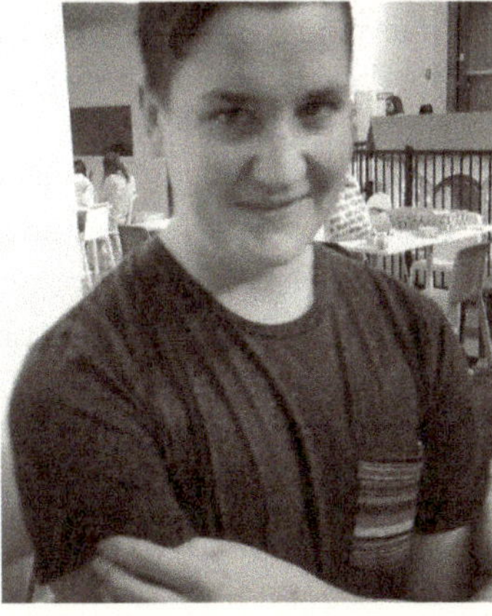

That was one of the last conversations I had with Ty.

In what turned out to be the last week of his life, Ty and I had transitioned from being two young boys playing backyard cricket and footy, wrestling in the lounge room, to organising dinners and beers during the week, going out to nightclubs, talking about girls and sharing confidences.

You don't know what you've got until it's gone. This resonates so much for me when it comes to my relationship with Ty. In that week we'd gone from brothers to mates. We were having grown up conversations. Dad had just bought him a new car to learn how to drive, he had a new tattoo, and if there had been a tomorrow, he would have started a building apprenticeship with a local business in Hobart.

He was a bloody man now. But Ty and I only had one week of that transition, and there's no way I'll ever get it back again. That loss is incredibly difficult for me to deal with.

All we could see was Ty about to go through a life transition, from childhood to adulthood and independence. This stage comes for us all. For some it happens early, for some it happens later. It's a challenging but exciting time.

What we didn't think was that transitions can be a scary thing. Or that Ty might be finding it challenging. We didn't think that he was anything but excited about this next chapter of life. And we certainly didn't consider he might not be coping with his feelings or thoughts, or that it would lead to such a decision.

Clearly Ty had more on his mind in the last few weeks of his life than just learning to drive and fitting in with new colleagues.

CHAPTER 5

The aftermath

I FINALLY got back to Dad's place that night, completely exhausted. I needed to sleep. I jumped into bed with my hoodie on to warm up and relieve my sciatica. After walking around barefoot in the cold wearing just shorts and a T-shirt, it had started to play up.

I felt completely numb going downstairs to my cold bedroom. The intensity of the feelings and thoughts over the last hours had left me drained. But still in shock, thoughts and memories and images turning over in my head, I just couldn't sleep. I remember checking Facebook and finding hundreds of messages sending love, hoping I was OK, and offering kind words about Ty.

Restless, I wandered back upstairs. I felt absolute emptiness. Dad was up, sitting at the kitchen bench with his head in his hands. Koula and Grandma were there too, having teas and coffees.

I don't recall saying much, just thinking to myself, "What the fuck do we do now?"

My back was still aching and I felt frustrated at feeling physical pain when I was dealing with something outside of myself that was so much bigger.

It was a cold morning but I needed fresh air and to move my body. I rugged up and walked on my own along the river. I couldn't stop crying. I just kept whispering to myself, over and over, 'This isn't happening, this can't have happened, not to Ty'. He was the last person in my world who I thought would die. How could he not be here anymore? How is it possible I would never see him again? I walked for an hour, zigzagging across the road to avoid people's stares as I wept.

Sahar had arrived early, telling her family she was off to work. My mates didn't go to work, and instead came round to be with me. By mid-morning, the garage door was up and there were cars everywhere. We sat around in the garage in a big circle. Someone went out to get food and beer. Friends and family sat around as Dad said a few words. He thanked everyone for coming over and how we couldn't believe what had happened.

They stayed with us all day. Mum and Dad had barely spoken since they had separated, but they did manage to spend time together. Mum and Glenn with Dad and Koula, sitting down having a drink in the garage — but it took the worst of circumstances to make it happen.

That day is foggy in my memory. I did a lot of mindless standing around, floating between discussions and groups of people as if I was outside of my body. I was restless and numb. I kept thinking about the normal day I should have been living. I should have been at work, getting Subway or bagging out my friends in our group message. Instead, I was here in this nightmare. How could it be possible? I'd get to talking about something else and my mind would relax, but would be jolted back to the reality that Ty wasn't with us. It still hadn't sunk in. I broke down again and again that day.

For Sahar, the loss of Ty opened up another issue. Because we were still only a new couple and hadn't told her family, she didn't know what she was going to say. She had been living two lives. I knew she wanted to be there for me, but how on earth was she going to return home in tears and explain what had happened? In the end, she called her cousin to explain the situation. They cried and made a plan for the short-term. That night at Sahar's parents', they used Jenna's name instead. Her mother, who had never have seen her daughter so upset, was able to comfort her without any complicated questions.

She worried about me that night, so Duck and Timmy stayed over. We took a photo of the three of us lying on the bed and texted it to her, just to let her know I was doing OK.

THE NEXT MORNING, Koula's cousin Alex, a funeral director, arrived to start organising Ty's funeral. It was weird to be sitting around the kitchen table with Mum, Glenn, Dad and Koula in the same room. It had been a long time since they had shared each other's company.

We spent a couple of hours discussing the venue and time, and eventually decided on Friday, January 18th 2013 as the day for the funeral. We arranged who would speak: Jenna, Dad, Glenn, and myself. Mum didn't feel that she could.

During that long conversation around the kitchen table, Alex, who was sitting next to me, asked "Did you notice Ty being down at all, Mitch?"

"No," I said, defensively, anger rising inside me. "We have no idea what happened."

He didn't say anything else, just reached out his arm, placing it on my shoulder as support.

It makes sense to me that in Alex's line of work as a funeral director he would deal with these situations more often than most. Other families may have been able to answer 'yes', but, in that moment, 'no' was the only answer I thought possible.

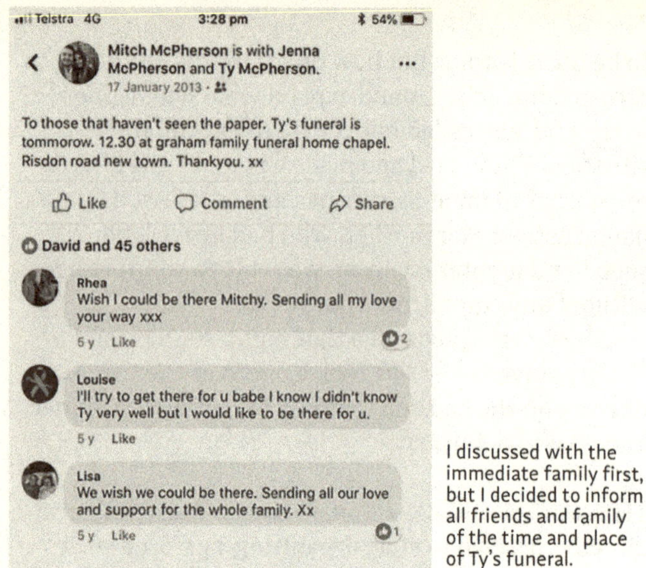

I discussed with the immediate family first, but I decided to inform all friends and family of the time and place of Ty's funeral.

THE DAYS IN THE LEAD UP to the funeral are a blur for me. We didn't know what to do except lounge around and stare into space.

When I look back on losing Ty, one thing I remember vividly is the support that rallied around us. I remember the number of people who gathered in the front yard at Mum's to support us on the night. I remember looking at my phone, receiving so many texts. People were calling in all the time, dropping off meals, tidying up, offering their condolences and love. Anything to help ease our burden.

The night before the funeral, a group of my friends from Melbourne arrived at home. Ben, Sam, Julien and Kristy-Lea had been on the phone to me all week, and it was an emotional moment to see their cab pull up. I needed people around to distract me, because being alone with my thoughts was too hard. I knew I'd be drawn into a black hole of fear and sadness and guilt, and I couldn't face it yet.

Ben, my best mate, stayed the night and slept on a spare mattress we had dragged downstairs onto the floor in my room. We stayed awake for a long time everyone had gone to bed. Through the darkest hours of my life, not being able to have my girlfriend with me, it was Ben who eased small amounts of the incredible pain I was feeling, and kept me from falling into that black hole.

SOMEHOW THE WEEK PASSED and Friday came, the day of Ty's funeral.

I finished writing my speech as we were getting ready to go, along with a note for Ty that I wanted to place with his body. We had all been told we could write something and leave it in his casket to stay with him forever. I can't remember exactly what I put in my note, but I filled an entire page of a cheap lined notepad. I remember trying to tell Ty all the things I'd miss doing with him. I asked him why he had done this and how he had gotten here. There was anger in the note – my own fear and guilt coming out. But it was mostly messages of reassurance and love.

Looking back I was very lucky to have so much support flowing in. A Facebook post was a great way to let everyone out there know that the support wasn't going unnoticed.

Telstra 4G
3:28 pm
54%
Mitch McPherson
16 January 2013 ·
I'm sorry I haven't replied to everyone. But the messages and calls I've received is overwhelming. Thankyou.
Like
Comment
Share
Sahar and 110 others
Garry
i have just seen it Mitch please accept my deepest Sympathy for your loss
5 y Like
Mitch McPherson
Cheers gaz xx
5 y Like
Jane
xxxxxx
5 y Like

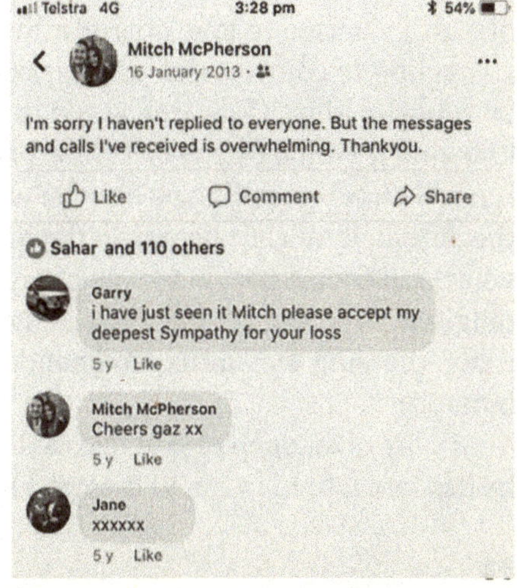

Telstra 4G
3:27 pm
54%
Mitch McPherson ▶ Ty McPherson
19 January 2013 · Kingston Beach, TAS ·
I love you my man. And I miss you so much already.
Like
Comment
Sally and 36 others

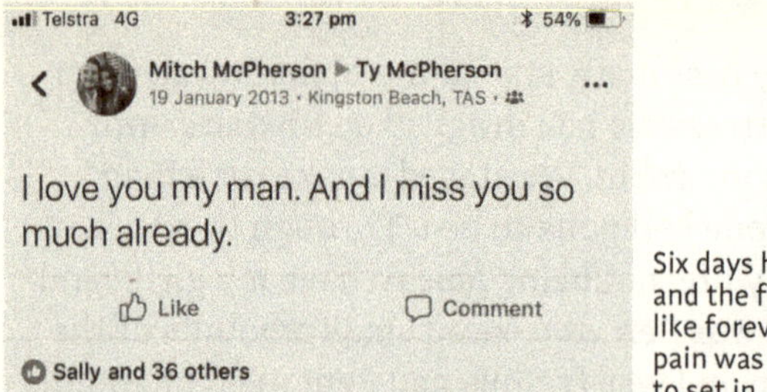

Six days had gone by, and the funeral seemed like forever away. The pain was really starting to set in.

We got to the funeral home early, as we had been told we could spend some time with Ty before the service. I was with family and had arranged to meet Sahar, Ben and Timmy. We all hugged outside before making our way into the funeral home.

Inside there were a few quiet greetings as everyone arrived. We started toward the back where Ty was lying behind the curtain in an open casket. Suddenly, Timmy turned to me and said he couldn't see Ty; that as much as he wanted to, it was just something he didn't want to face. He stayed behind whilst the rest of us headed in together.

I had thought a lot about Ty's body that week. I thought about that image of him, lying still and cold in the lounge room that night. I thought of him being at the morgue, on a steel tray in a wall somewhere, like on TV. I used to love horror movies, but I was struggling to connect those images of dead bodies with my brother. I knew I wanted to see him again, knowing it would be the last time. I recall Alex, the funeral director, telling us how he would dress Ty on the day. Insignificant details in the grand scheme of what was happening, but I was clinging to anything tangible, anything I could make sense of. I felt some relief knowing Ty was in good hands before we laid him to rest.

Ty lay in an open casket dressed in the black suit he had worn to his year 10 formal. I placed the letter

I had written beside him, folded into a tiny square. I knelt down and held his hand. A crowd was jostling to see him. It was chaotic and emotional as we tried to process this being the last time we'd ever see Ty. Mum was sobbing uncontrollably, hunched over him. I said my goodbyes and backed away, but kept going back to have another moment with Ty — to touch him, hold his hand, rub his hair.

We all stayed as long as we could until it was time to get proceedings under way. We sat together as a family and the service was packed. I wasn't surprised that nearly 1400 people turned up to say goodbye to Ty.

As we sat there waiting for the service to begin, I noticed Mum, a mix of sadness, anger, unease and fear on her face. She looked like she was about to explode, and needed to get it together.

I got up from my seat and moved about two metres to my left where Mum was sitting. I leaned over and put my head to Mum's.

"Mum, Ty wouldn't want you to be angry, just relax, OK, and do it for Ty."

It took her a moment, but she calmed down and began breathing slowly again.

Lots of Ty's friends were sitting together and I remember feeling so sad that they had lost such a good friend. They were so young themselves, how were they processing this?

Shortly after, the curtains were drawn and the casket was closed behind them. We watched on as Ty's casket was wheeled to the front of the church. We were all sitting there, hushed, waiting for the service to begin when Ty's football coach walked to the front of the room and handed Ty's footy jumper to Glenn. Football was important to Ty, and he prided himself on being a good player and part of a team. I decided to do something with it, so I stood up, took the guernsey from Glenn and draped it over the casket.

I don't remember much of what the celebrant said. Sadness and grief clouded my focus and shut out much of what was going on around me. But I do remember him reminding us to grateful that Ty had touched our lives, and to do what Ty would have wanted: "to smile, open our eyes, love and go on".

Dad gave the first tribute and he was struggling to breathe through his tears.

Finally, he said, "I'm Tig's Dad ..." There was the longest pause. In those simple words, it hit home that Tig was no longer with us, as a son, as a brother, as a mate. As Tig.

"We're overwhelmed at the show of love for Tig and support for his family," he continued. He talked about Tig's beautiful heart and soul, his sense of humour, how he always had a cheeky grin.

"To me it always looked like he was up to no good," said Dad, trying to find some levity in the moment.

"Tig," said Dad, his voice cracking, "I'm ripped apart. Goodbye son, talk to you soon."

Glenn, Jenna and Emmanuel spoke next, sharing their memories of Ty and reflecting on their relationships with him. Glenn reminded every person in the crowd: 'Never stop talking to your families. You don't realise how gut wrenching this is.'

When it came to my turn, I spoke about the week, the grief, how broken I felt, and about missing Ty. I'd written a poem and I could barely read through tears. When I sat down, Dad got up and gave me a big hug. He gave everyone a hug after they'd spoken.

"If there's any consolation," said our celebrant, "Ty will be forever young, handsome and 18."

For Sahar, it was the biggest, most emotional funeral she had ever attended. She kept thinking if only Ty was there to see how much people had cared about him.

Dad, Jenna, Emmanuel, Glenn, Pop and I carried out Ty's casket. I'll never forget how heavy it was. Jenna was in front of me and I could see her really struggling, battling to hold it. At one stage, it became so heavy, even I felt I couldn't hold it much longer. Finally, we made it to the hearse and laid the casket inside it. The burial site was only a five-minute drive away and we invited anyone to come if they wanted to.

About 70 people came to the short but sweet burial ceremony, and it was nice that it didn't last long. Ty's casket was lowered into the ground and it was time for me to release two white doves into the sky. When I knelt down and opened the lid of the box containing the doves, one panicked and left a big runny bird shit on my suit jacket. I was too busy looking for something to wipe my suit with and missed them taking flight to freedom and the blue sky beyond. They were meant as a symbol of Ty's soul, two doves carrying his spirit above us, watching over us. I felt desperately sad that I'd missed them. But the mood soon turned to laughter when people saw what had happened, and it brought a lighter moment to the occasion.

As the ceremony came to its close, the silence was deafening. We dropped different coloured roses on top of Ty's casket, then a handful of dirt each. As each rose and handful of dirt was thrown onto the casket, the silence was replaced by wailing. We couldn't hold it in any longer.

In burying and saying goodbye to a loved one, there are stages where you are frozen, lost in a powerful, overwhelming emotion that shuts out everything around you. Then all of a sudden, it's like you wake from a daydream and reality hits you all over again, as intense as the first time. I moved through these stages over and over at the funeral, leaving me hollow and exhausted.

At Ty's wake, Sahar was struck by the different approaches to dealing with grief. She hadn't experienced a Western funeral before and was shocked to be around seemingly happy people when they had just lived through the worst week of their lives. She couldn't understand why people were laughing, making jokes and drinking when Ty was no longer with us. All the funerals she had attended previously were from her Syrian culture, where there is a lengthy grieving stage when someone passes. You wear black, there is no drinking, people stop watching TV or doing anything that would bring them happiness. It is a period of ultimate sadness.

There is no right or wrong way to grieve, and perhaps a period of deep mourning allows us to truly experience and embrace our grief. But we desperately needed to find some light to help us through this dark time. So we laughed, joked and drank together to remind ourselves of better times and find some escape from the weight of our sadness.

Death and grief were things I was unfamiliar with. With my family and close friends all still around, the only experiences of death I had were distant. A guy I played footy with died in a car accident. Duck's Dad died from cancer. Ben's Pop died from meningococcal. Those moments were sad, but they weren't enough to have ever made me sit down and think about how would I cope if those losses happened to me. I had never thought about what I would do or to whom I would turn if I lost someone close. It had never even occurred to me to be ready for it.

CHAPTER 6

Time standing still

I KEPT telling myself once the funeral was over I would be OK again. I was convinced that if I just got through that day then the hardest part would be over and things would get easier.

The sad reality was that after the funeral, it got much worse. People who'd visited from interstate flew home, friends and family all went back to work, and whilst people still thought of Ty, life for them kept on moving. My world, however, had stopped. I didn't feel I had anything to go back to, or that I could rebuild. Not with the loss I was reeling from. My mates still rang me every day, family were calling in now and then, but they couldn't be there all the time. They had their own lives and their own concerns, and rightly so. But at a certain point, support from family and friends can't help you avoid or escape the grief that's inside of you. After the whirlwind of Ty's death, its aftermath and the funeral, I was left to face that from within.

How do you live again when your little brother has gone? How do you concentrate on anything? How do you ever find happiness or joy in everyday life again? Finding the answers to these questions proved to be the biggest challenge yet.

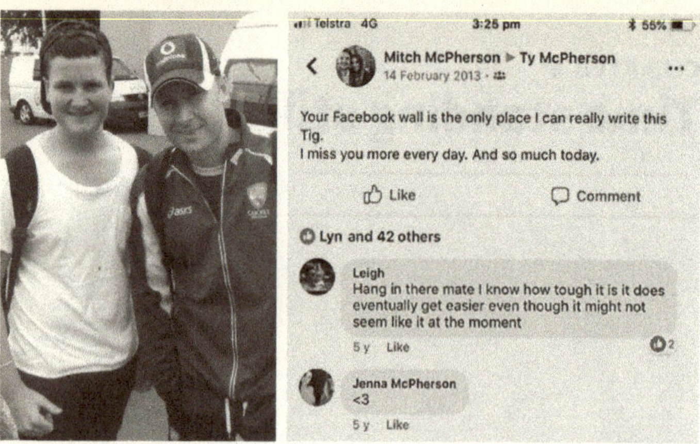

I show this photo of Ty with former Australian cricket captain Michael Clarke as part of my PowerPoint presentation. It shows so much of who Ty was and his character — I love it!

Looking back, I recall that being able to express love for Ty on social media was a huge outlet for me.

AFTER THE FUNERAL, I took a week off work. People were telling me that it was good to go back to work when someone dies and not isolate yourself in your bedroom; that it's best to get routine back in your life. But I couldn't. There was no way I could function and interact with people so soon. Scott said he'd let me start fresh the following week. He paid me for the week I had missed, and told me he would cover the upcoming week off too. This was incredibly kind. I had no holidays banked up and my finances were starting to add to my stress.

Australia was playing cricket that week at Blundstone Arena, and it was a good distraction to see the game, doing normal things again with Emmanuel and Dad. But everything I did seemed to highlight the brutal fact that Ty wasn't around to go to the cricket or the gym or go for a drive. My brother wasn't with us any more. Ty was dead. I continued to ask myself how the hell that was even possible.

I thought about it constantly, my brain was going a million miles an hour trying to process how this could be. One thing I couldn't stop dwelling on was the moment I spent with Ty at the funeral home. My final memory of my active, bright, fun-loving little brother was of him lying there, motionless, cold and pale-faced, in the suit he had worn to his school formal. I found myself slipping into an endless loop thinking about it, and in the process, bringing myself to tears. I knew it was unhealthy to focus on this distressing thought when I had so many fond memories of Ty to draw upon, but my mind wouldn't let me forget it. I tried to distract myself, but fell hard back to earth each time I confronted the present. I wish I could remember what I did that week ... but I just can't.

TWO WEEKS after Ty's death, I knew I had to get routine back into my life. So I picked myself up and went back to work. But I had a lot of breakdowns doing my job that week, and on one occasion had to go home. Most days I was driving past the cemetery where we buried Ty, and this proved to be a battle for me.

Scott took me aside on that first morning back to work. He told me he would put me with one of my favourite colleagues, Jayden, because we worked well together. We had played footy together, and Jayden had also known Ty. Not only that, he had a brother five years younger and he might be able to understand and empathise with how I was feeling.

Working with Jayden helped me through those early days. We'd often go and visit Ty's grave. We'd take a Subway roll for lunch, and a Powerade or a V can for Tig, and sit there and talk. Jayden said when he found out about Ty, all he could think about was how he would feel if it were his younger brother.

After a couple of weeks, I felt I needed to work on my own again. It got harder from there, and at times I felt like I was going backwards. There wasn't a day

I didn't struggle. I can't remember what I did to find the strength I needed to get out of bed, go to work, to live my life. I certainly wasn't engaged in it, I was just going through the motions.

Some nights I'd simply go and sit in Ty's room. Dad had made it into a shrine. He'd cleaned it, but we didn't want to touch it, not even change the sheets. I spent so many days in there, sitting on his bed and crying, just missing him so much. Eventually Dad and Koula moved, and Ty's things got packed up. Mum is still in the same house, and she swears she will never move. When Mum gets upset, she'll often go into Ty's room and do exactly what we all need to do sometimes – just cry and grieve.

Mum and Glenn turned their garage into a shrine as well. They printed out every photo they had of Ty and pinned them to the walls as a way of dealing with their loss. Those photos remain there to this day and cover every wall.

That's how the first six months passed after losing Ty. I had no aspirations of starting anything new. We just had to adjust to life without Ty. There were a lot of awful days, with tears and sadness as we navigated our loss.

Listening to music helped. I listened to a lot of music and a few songs got played on repeat. "Mirrors" by Justin Timberlake was my favourite for a while. I still love that song, but it reminds me so much of the time when we lost Ty, and I have to be in the right headspace to listen to it. If I'm not, I can get into a panic because I know what it can trigger.

Mum worked at the Metro bus company, which offered counselling to employees and their families. I went once, but I found more strengthen and comfort in talking to family and friends, breaking down in front of Sahar and Dad, and having a hug rather than talking to a counsellor. The connection wasn't the same as what I could get from someone who knew Ty, so I went once and never went back. The irony is, now I preach about the importance of seeking help and trying more than once to find the right fit. Maybe it would have helped had I stuck with it. I certainly see the value in it today.

Losing a family member is one of the hardest things in life, but losing one to suicide feels harder. The guilt you are saddled with is relentless and intense. You can spend an eternity questioning what happened, blaming yourself for not doing more. Feeling ashamed you didn't see the signs, or wondering if you'd been better would it have changed anything. And there is anger too. Anger at the person for leaving you like this, for not believing that you cared for them.

This was especially true for Dad. He had spent Tig's last day with him. He had dropped him off and Tig had told him, "I'll be right". Dad could never have imagined that the next thing his youngest boy would do was end his life.

Dad and I often golfed in the summertime. After we lost Ty I asked Dad if he wanted to play a game with me and the boys sometime. I was taken aback when he gave a flat out no. He told me he didn't ever want to play golf again, because the last game he'd played was with Ty. He wanted to keep that memory special.

SADLY, not long after losing Ty, we lost Nan and Pop. Both to cancer. Although I was extremely close to Nan and Pop, losing Ty to suicide was a thousand times harder to deal with than losing them to natural causes.

Their deaths left me with two big holes in my heart. I couldn't have loved them any more if I tried;

they really were two beautiful people. They were the heartbeat of Mum's side of the family that kept them together.

Pop passed away about a year and a half after Ty, and Nan died within the same year. Pop had become ill with cancer and ended up in hospital. It wasn't good and we all knew he wasn't going to make it. Sadly I missed his funeral. I feel I never got to say an official goodbye. That hurts, given how much he loved me.

Soon after, we watched Nan slowly deteriorate. She started to lose her wit and her functioning. Nan had always been 'go go go', so to see her needing a carer most days and relying on my Auntie Maritza for day-to-day things was tough. It all seemed to happen so quickly with Nan, and all of a sudden she too was in the hospital's cancer ward, and her days were limited.

Looking back on the loss of my two grandparents, I know that the sadness and sense of loss I felt for them was nothing like the total, all-consuming grief I felt at losing Ty. It made me feel like a heartless prick that their loss did not devastate me more. Why didn't I ache more for them? Why didn't I mourn them more? Did I not love them enough? Had I lost my capacity to feel?

I realise now that I'm not a prick at all. I'm not heartless and it doesn't mean I didn't love my grandparents enough. What it means is that I've been affected by suicide and that my heart has been rocked by something much more traumatic. Suicide changes you as a person. It numbs feeling and makes everything around it seem small.

Nan and Pop will always hold a special place in my heart. I miss them so much, but also know they are looking down on me with pride. Nan will forever be singing to the ends of the earth, "Oh, look at my boy".

CHAPTER 7

Missing the signs

FOR WEEKS after losing Ty people would ask, "Were there any signs that Ty was struggling?" My knee-jerk reaction was always, "No, no way". Again and again I explained that Ty was the last person I imagined could be battling, that he was happy and ready to face his future.

It was a long time before I started to think more deeply about Ty in the lead up to his death, about the possibility of him not being himself. There were so many unanswered questions, and I became fixated on what took my brother away. I read as much as I could about mental ill-health and suicide, what can happen to a person and how they might act if they are struggling with mental health issues or thoughts of suicide.

I needed to find out what makes someone take their own life.

I know now that there are no definite answers about what led Ty to his actions. Suicide is extremely complex, and there's never usually one reason. But in trying to find these answers, I finally had to acknowledge my undeniable ignorance. How could I have lived my life without ever thinking that mental illness or suicide could touch me or the ones I love? How could I have thought these issues, which affect so many of us, were so unimportant?

As time went by, and after many conversations with my family, Sahar, and my brothers' friends, I reflected on the moments I had seen Ty, or times I spent with him before he passed. Sadly, I was starting to realise that when I told people I didn't see Ty showing signs that he wasn't OK, I was wrong.

It became apparent to me that Ty was showing plenty of signs that he wasn't quite right; that he was struggling. But we as a family, and in particular me as his brother and his best friend, failed to recognise these signs, and didn't bother to act on them and ask if everything was all right.

ONE SIGN is so obvious to me now.

I have never met anyone more excited by dinnertime. Ty was like Usain Bolt, literally running as fast as he could to the dinner table of an evening. Nothing else mattered to Tig when there was food on offer. He would get to the kitchen table, grab a knife and fork and all but start banging them on the table, just so excited to get stuck into his meal.

At Dad's place, if we weren't at footy or soccer training or out with friends, we tried to have dinner together. It was our family way of catching up, checking in and enjoying some time together. Ty in particular was always vocal at the dinner table, chattering away, joking, bagging us out and driving the conversation.

But in those last couple of weeks, I recall there were three, four, even five nights when Ty didn't join us for dinner. A meal was served, someone would shout out that dinner was ready, but he just didn't answer or told us he wasn't hungry. Instead of rushing to join us like he usually would, he stayed away and kept himself in his room. On those evenings, we heard him come out of his room, go to the toilet, brush his teeth, but other than that he didn't interact with anyone.

With what I know now about mental ill-health, those moments should have been alarm bells for us – but sadly they weren't. One of us should have gone into his bedroom and checked in with him. One of us should have sent him a text and asked is everything OK. But like a lot of families, we just assumed, he's 18, he's just having a quiet night and wants to be by himself. Not one of us went in and asked that question, "Are you OK"?

I understand that kids grow up. That with age comes less interaction with parents and siblings, and more independence. If it had only been one occasion when Ty hadn't joined us for dinner, I wouldn't look back on this situation so harshly. But I can see now there was a clear, sudden change in Ty's behaviour, and I want to scream it from the rooftops – that kind of change needs to be noticed.

THERE WERE other signs.

Four days before Ty took his own life, I was driving toward home. It was about 4pm. Ty got out a lot and mingled with friends after school or his part time work, and was notorious for sending a text or making a call for one of us to come and pick him up.

I was cruising in my ute, still 10 minutes from home, when I spotted Ty on the side of the road, walking in the same direction.

I pulled up next to him, wound down the window and cleared my things off the front seat.

"Hey Tig, hop in," I said. "I'll give you a lift."

Ty looked at me, peering through the window.

"No, I'm okay. I'm happy to walk."

"Are you joking?" I said, surprised he didn't want to get in and come home with me as he usually would.

"No, I'm all good. I'll see you at home," Ty said.

"Righto," I said.

I wound up the window and drove off.

I will never forget the night I remembered that encounter with Tig. It was some weeks after he died. I was sitting at home on the couch with Sahar, watching TV, trying to keep my mind off things.

All of a sudden, my mind took me back to that afternoon. I broke down and fell into a heap on the floor. I remembered how I'd asked Ty if he wanted a lift, how he'd declined, and how I'd just driven off. But what I remembered most was looking back at him in the rear view mirror as I drove away. Head down, shuffling steps, walking so slowly it would have taken him another half hour to get home. He was clearly someone who wasn't in the right headspace. Someone who had something on his mind.

Ty would usually jump on the bonnet, jump through the window of the car to get a lift home. Lock me in for that game of cricket, have a laugh and tell me about his day. On that occasion, he did the opposite and I didn't think twice. I just left him there.

It was, and continues to be, a moment I struggle with. I wish that I had gotten out of the car and walked with him, asked him what was wrong, and reassured him that I was there for him. I wish I had acted differently that afternoon.

THERE ARE PLENTY of things I have battled with since losing Tig. So many "what if" moments that have played over in my mind. What did I miss, what could I have done differently. What if I had been better or more attentive or more supportive? Would it have changed anything?

One in particular hits me the hardest, and has taken me down some lonely roads and sleepless nights. My eyes still fill with tears when I speak about it. Sometimes, I fear it will just take me over.

It was Sunday, the night before Ty passed away. He was spending the night with us, and going off in the morning with Dad to run errands. Every evening I'd do the rounds, say goodnight to everyone and make my way downstairs to my bedroom.

I showered, brushed by teeth, came out of the bathroom and headed into to Ty's room to say goodnight. His bedroom door was shut, normal at this hour, so it wasn't anything alarming. I busted my way in, as every big brother should.

"Good night Tig," I said. "I'll see you tomorrow."

Ty was lying on his stomach with his hat on backwards, playing on his phone. He didn't answer. I guess I thought he just didn't hear me, so I stepped in a bit closer.

"Tig, night, see you tomorrow," I said, a bit louder this time.

Finally, he half-turned his head towards me.

"Night ..." he mumbled.

"Catch you later", I shouted, pulling his door shut, and heading to bed.

I never saw my little brother again.

That moment is incredibly hard to live with. Not only was it the last time I saw or spoke to Ty, but my inaction in that moment is the greatest regret of my life. Ty's face that night was ashen and tearful. He was lying there with a mountain of issues on his mind and in his heart.

Instead of concern, I didn't think anything of it when he half looked at me, mumbled, and just said, "Night". I thought he was a bit grumpy. I thought what a sook – what could possibly be wrong with him. Is he worried about going to work? He's bloody 18! He's got the world at his feet!

I knew Ty. I knew that he would have been desperate for me to notice everything wasn't right. Desperate for me to ask if everything was OK. He would have been struggling to make that first move and tell me he was in pain.

I wish every day that I'd sat on the edge of his bed and told him that it's OK to cry, to lean on me. I wish I'd given him a hug and listened to what was going on for him. I wish I had taken him out to chat with Dad or Koula, and made him see that his family were there to support him and help him through this dark time he was facing.

For a lot of brothers that conversation would be bloody tough. Letting your guard down, showing you care, and exposing your softer side is something us blokes aren't good at. But I would give anything in the world to have that moment again. If I just knew the importance of not hiding your feelings. If I knew that it was OK to not be OK, and that it's helpful to tell someone about it. Ty needed connection, support and reassurance. He needed to know we loved him. If I'd given that to him, would he still be with us today?

I believe we didn't see the signs in Ty's behaviour because of our ignorance about mental ill-health. Ty's friends didn't notice a change in him – probably because they saw him in happy times, hanging out and enjoying life – whereas I caught him in those times when he was on his own, in bed about to go to sleep, or walking home at the end of the day. In those situations, it should have been obvious that something was wrong.

I also believe, after learning a lot more about mental health, that a good conversation at that moment between brothers could have saved Ty's life. I don't think he had been dealing with an untreated mental health issue like depression. I don't believe he was in a deep hole. I believe he was on the edge and needed someone to grab him and pull him back.

Australian men are raised to be tough, to be providers for their family, a bit larrikin, and to not let anything get them down. I'm sure I always thought like that. I was a tradie, I played footy, liked having a laugh with my mates ... If I ever had a shitty day I'd put on a brave face and keep it myself. I suppose I expected my brother to do the same. So I did nothing.

I still feel that I failed in my role as big brother – to look out for and protect Ty. But in my young adult mind, I didn't know it was my role to play. I failed to learn about an issue that is very real. I failed to see that mental ill-health was happening under our own roof. If I'd had the courage to challenge those 'Australian man' norms, or had sat in on some mental health training, I wonder if I'd feel less guilty.

Even though I still struggle with guilt and unanswered questions, one thing I have finally learned is that if somebody decides to take their own life, that is their decision. People kept telling me it wasn't my fault, but it took me a long time to believe it. I still have to work hard to believe it and accept that it was Ty's decision.

AFTER SIX MONTHS, we were all still asking ourselves, "Why Ty?" Why did he, of all people, take his own life? We had learned about a few small factors that may have built up and contributed to Ty becoming suicidal – work, girl troubles, a few different stresses here and there. He was also hungover and tired. Or maybe we missed something bigger. We'll never know for sure, but I truly don't think it was much more than that. Perhaps it was that simple – an impulsive decision, a spur-of-the-moment action when he wasn't handling things or couldn't see a way out.

And there was no coming back from that decision.

When we put together the final hours of Ty's life, we learned that after Dad had dropped Ty off at Mum's, someone saw him walk up the street. We have no idea where he went to or what he did, but he returned home not long after that.

There were no other explanations, nothing else that could have been a clue. If there had been a build up and he'd thought about it the night before or during the time he'd spent with Dad, maybe there would have been more detail in the letter. But to us it seems he didn't put any more thought into it than that moment at home.

I have never wanted to go into detail as to how Ty took his life. I obviously know, but it's detail I need not ever think about.

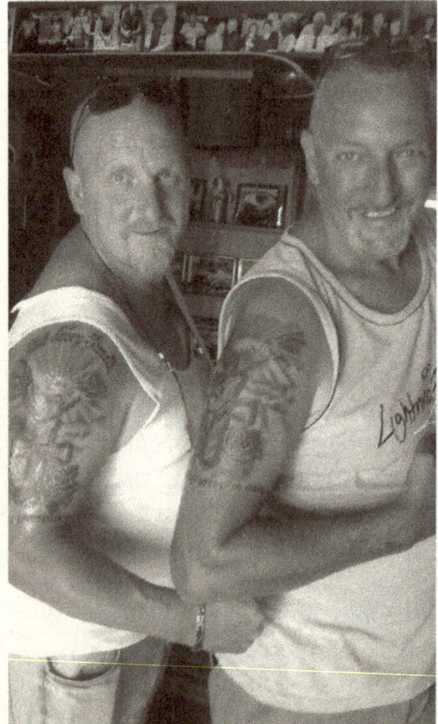

My Dad Dale and my Step Dad Glenn both got matching tattoos to always remember Ty by. It was the first tattoo that either of them had ever had.

CHAPTER 8

Ignorance can be fatal

WHEN I WAS just out of primary school, we lived in a Hobart suburb called Oakdowns. It was one of the nicest, newest houses we had ever lived in, and the last home I had with both Mum and Dad before they separated.

I used to knock around with Nick, a boy who lived in the same street. He was a fun guy, a couple of years younger than me, great at sport and popular with the girls. We used to have heaps of fun riding our bikes around the bush together. How good it was to finish school, get home, and know that down the road there was someone just as keen as you to jump on a bike and go exploring.

I don't remember much about Nick, but there is one event that has always stuck in my mind. One day, Nick and I were hitting a tennis ball outside my house with tennis racquets, talking rubbish more than likely, when a woman walked past with a big German Shepherd on a lead, barking like mad at the tennis ball I had in my hand. They moved within arm's reach of me, the dog dragging the woman closer. "Does he bite?" I asked. At that moment, the dog lunged at me, dragging me down by my shoulder onto the road.

It was quite a panic as the three of us tried to drag the dog off me. Thankfully, it only lasted a few seconds and eventually he let go, leaving a hole in my jacket and a trace of blood on my right shoulder where the teeth had pierced my skin. I still have a tiny tooth mark scar and a lifelong fear of German Shepherds. My parents were out so Nick's mum phoned the local GP to ask about my latest tetanus shot, which it turned out, I didn't need. After getting cleaned up, I jumped back on my bike and got on with my day.

When Mum and Dad separated we moved away from Oakdowns, leaving behind my last memories of our family all together, as well as my friendship with Nick. I'm sure it was disappointing at the time, but at that age, you meet new people every day and we moved house quite a bit, so I don't recall it being a huge drama.

Years later, when I was about 20, we got news that Nick had killed himself. He left his parents behind on their own, with no other children. 'Suicide' was barely a word mentioned in my life then, so it was a surprise to hear it when it happened. I hadn't seen Nick for a few years, but I remember reflecting on his death, trying to fathom how someone comes to that decision. How does someone with so much going for them not want to live anymore? How can they do that to their parents? All I remember is not being able to understand it in the slightest.

I recall talking to Ty about Nick, about how he had killed himself and how sad it was. I remember Ty asking, "How could anyone do that?" At that stage in Ty's life, he had never felt pain. He hadn't lived long enough to understand that one day he might feel how Nick did.

Our conversation that afternoon did do one thing. It showed how ignorant we were, how much knowledge we lacked on such an important issue. We were two young men, brothers, discussing suicide, a topic that we knew very little about. In fact, there was a bit of judgment about how Nick could knowingly leave his parents on their own, heartbroken, without any other kids. We couldn't understand. Ty had no idea his life would end the same way as Nick's. And I had no idea that I would come to feel the exact pain Nick's family felt.

That conversation with Ty ended too soon. I should have known a lot more about suicide and how it could affect us. I wish that I had taken that conversation further but I didn't understand and I didn't have the words. I could have said to my little brother, "I am here for you if you are battling", or "Make sure you have a chat if you're in a bad space".

But I never did. If I had known what to say to Ty, if I had got him to talk to me if he was ever feeling down, might that have saved his life? Did my ignorance play a part in his death?

This is why I became so passionate about talking to people about suicide. To educate and to challenge that ignorance and that stigma. Because in the future there will be more brothers driving in a car talking about "that guy" that took his own life, or parents noticing their child is just one per cent off, and I pray that they might know the right thing to say in that moment. If they do, they may not end up feeling what I feel, every day, when I think of my late brother.

I am confident that my little brother didn't speak to us about his battles was because of the fear he would be seen as weak or different. He was 18 years old with plenty going for him. I know he would have thought about ways to open up and share the painful thoughts running through his mind. But fear of looking weak or strange puts up a wall for people who might need to talk about their feelings or thoughts.

It is only in the last couple of years that high profile people have started speaking publicly about their struggles with their mental health. It's fantastic that these individuals have had the courage to name it up and talk about it. I have no doubt that the likes of footballer Buddy Franklin, billionaire businessman James Packer, and netball player Sharni Layton, opening up about their own personal battles is saving lives. They are making these conversations easier in schools, workplaces and sporting clubs across the country. They are showing us that even the best of us can struggle, that mental health issues don't discriminate, and that it's OK to not be OK. I hope this means we are moving toward a social place where people who are struggling feel like they can speak out, and those of us around them are comfortable supporting them.

While it's good we are hearing more about mental health issues, unfortunately we hear more and more about suicide deaths. Michael Hutchence from INXS, actor Robin Williams, chef Anthony Bourdain and singer Chester Bennington from Linkin Park have all, among others, sadly taken their lives in the past decade. Big names are role models for all of us, and in particular our young people. Hearing these tragic stories should be a reminder for all to challenge those misconceptions we have about mental health and suicide, and try to make a difference.

The world is changing, and we are starting to talk more comfortably about mental health and suicide instead of just thinking that it is someone else's problem. Maybe we all realise suicide is far too common and we can no longer continue to sweep it under the rug. But as a community and a culture, we're still navigating how we talk about these issues publicly.

After Ty, I now see the terrible stigma associated with mental health and suicide when it's reported in the media. News bulletins will report on it, but will still shy away from naming it up as 'suicide'. Reporters will avoid using the word, instead saying, "There were no suspicious circumstances" even when it is blatantly obvious the person took their own life. Instead, the story ends with, "If you or someone you know is struggling, contact Lifeline on 13 11 14."

For me, naming it is of critical importance. We don't need to know details like names or means or locations. There are important reasons for not glorifying or sensationalising the circumstances. But if we want to get serious about breaking down barriers when it comes to mental health and suicide, we need to confront it directly when we're given the chance. In my experience, people are truly unaware of the scale of the issue, and we need to acknowledge the reality of suicide if we are ever going to change it.

I wish I had known more about suicide when Ty died. But there was and continues to be so much social silence around the subject that keeps us in the dark. It is not a subject to be whispered about or covered up. Suicide prevention is truly everyone's business.

CHAPTER 9

Rebuilding

TY IS NEVER very far from my thoughts and sometimes my grief is triggered in unexpected ways.

One day I was leaving the physiotherapist when I noticed a young boy walking by. He was about ten years of age, a little on the chubby side, and he was wearing the same uniform as Ty when he was in primary school. He reminded me so much of Ty, and I couldn't help noticing that he looked sad.

I watched him walk into the service station before getting back to my car. He came out of the servo eating an ice cream and I watched him walk past again and up the road. A big part of me wanted to go up to him and ask him if everything was all right. I wanted to have a chat with him without looking like a creep. In the end I let him walk on and just sent a text to mum about what had happened.

There are moments like that when I see kids in the street who look down. I want to reassure them or give them a hug but I can't. To take action where I couldn't with Ty. I just hope they're finding out about our organisation or others, and are getting help if they're struggling.

FOR A WHILE, I shared how I was feeling through posts and poems on Facebook.

My phone was busy with texts and calls, for this I truly thank you all.
A day that I love and look forward to, just isn't as great without seeing you.
You would have been one of the first to ring, but now I just listen for your voice in the wind.

Milestones now aren't as great as before, but being with you now I truly adore.
On your deck into the view I stare, with my new favorite drop that we both now share.

As the day grows older it's becoming so true, that the gift I wanted just won't be you.
Miss you more than anything!

Cc's in heaven my boy Tig.

I had rejected counselling, but this was an outlet that served as my source of support, making me feel like I wasn't alone. I would also visit Tig's grave to find that connection, to feel closer to him. In those early days, I used to sit beside him, listen to sad songs through my headphones and let out lots of tears. Crying helped and I did that as often as I needed too.

The grave looked a bit sad there for a while. Although it meant the world to us, to anyone else it was just a pile of dirt with flowers resting on it. There was no headstone at that point. In the interim, Dad decided to build a blue and white timber box. He called it 'Tig's deck' and it made the space a bit nicer and much more welcoming.

It was the perfect reminder of my little brother and the cheeky grin he wore. We left a whiteboard with felt markers so people could leave a note for Ty if they wanted. It felt good to rock up and see messages from people who had been to visit him.

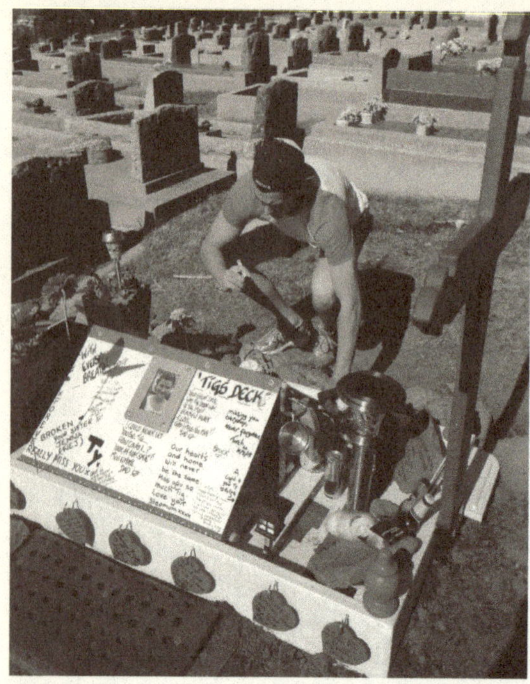

Writing messages to Ty each time we visited was a great way for us to all speak to him.

Ty's mates still visit on many occasions. It's heart-warming to see the bond his mates have and will forever hold onto.

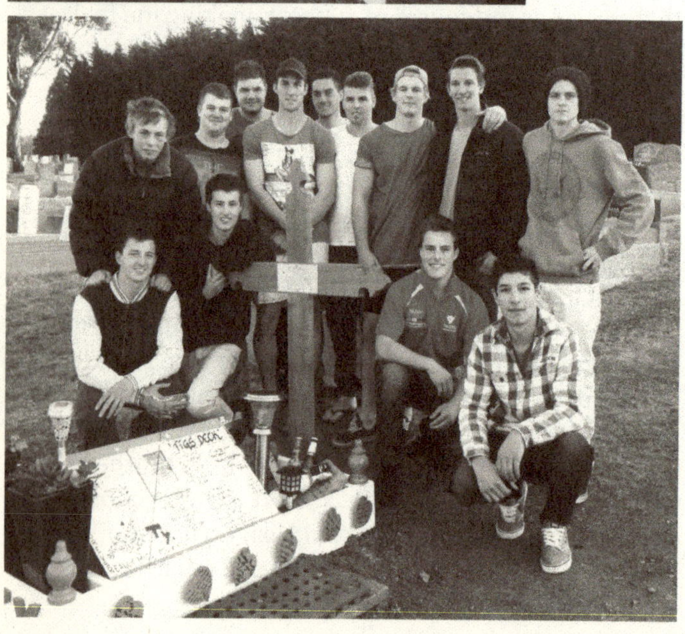

IN THOSE EARLY DAYS, Sahar's parents were still in the dark about me. We found ways to avoid telling them about us, which made life tough. I was grieving so much for my little brother, while at the same time wanting my girlfriend to be there so much more than she could. She wanted to be there for me, but it was just not possible. I was in a really dark place, but I didn't want to let her go. I knew deep down that I had to get it together. I would have to be in a better headspace to deal with what would come when they found out about our secret love for each other.

Inevitably, they found out — Tasmania is a small place, after all. As predicted, it didn't go down too well. Sahar's parents were upset and tried to keep her from seeing me. It couldn't have been worse timing. We had just started moving out of this phase of intense grief, becoming more stable and settled. It really threw me.

I have no idea where I found the courage to do this, but on the night they found out, I jumped in my car and drove to Sahar's Dad's shop. Sahar's father, Saad, along with his mother and five siblings, migrated to Australia with very little money to their name. They first lived in Greenacre in western Sydney in a near uninhabitable rental. As the years went by, they managed to save up enough money to buy a house of their own.

In 1979 they moved to Oatlands, a small country town in central Tasmania, where they bought a corner takeaway store. They saw an opportunity to work hard and be rewarded for it, and, at the same time, set up their children for a great future. It was a real family affair; the parents ran the shop while the kids helped out after school or during the school lunch hour. Saad attended the local high school and worked before and after school, and during lunchtime. They were the only ethnics living in Oatlands at the time and have never been forgotten by the town.

Later in life, Saad's parents bought a supermarket for their two youngest sons (one being Sahar's father). The locals used to refer to it as the 'Che Shop', named after Sahar's uncle, who was sadly killed in a car accident at the age of 18. Sahar's grandfather had made a Che Shop sign in Hawthorn colours in honour of Che, who was a massive Hawks fan.

Over the time that Sahar and I had been secretly going out, she told me so much about how her family came to Australia from Syria, and how their life had not always been the picture of success it is today. Now, finally, I found myself walking in to Sahar's father's store to meet him face to face.

Saad looked at me. Straight away he seemed to know who I was so I reached out to shake his hand.

"Hello Saad," I said. "I'm Mitch."

I had pictured her Dad as this big, scary man, the kind to have a baseball bat under the counter. But he couldn't have been more different. We shook hands. In a roundabout way, I told him that I loved his daughter, that she meant absolutely everything to me and I wanted to be a part of the family. He looked at me with warmth in his eyes.

"We'll work this out together," he said.

I always knew that I wanted to be with Sahar for the rest of my life. And I knew deep down that for me to fully become part of Sahar's life I would need to ask her to marry me. So I liaised with a local jeweller to have an engagement ring made, ready for the right moment. I was at a time in my life when I knew I was ready to marry and settle down. On November 29, 2014, almost two years after Ty's death, I decided to propose to Sahar.

The night before I went back to see Sahar's Dad at his store. This time it was to tell Saad that I had a ring, and that I was going to ask Sahar to marry me the very next day. Getting down on one knee and proposing is far from the traditional way Arabs signify their love. I wasn't really expecting Saad to jump for joy and show a huge amount of excitement about this news, but it still surprised me how totally relaxed he was.

"Yeah, yeah. That sounds good mate," he said. "I'll organise something at home in a couple of weeks".

Saad seemed more worried about closing up the shop than showing me some love for asking for his daughter's hand in marriage. I would come to know Sahar's father as the easiest-to-please man on the planet. Nothing seems to faze him; he is rarely stressed or troubled.

The next day I packed a surprise picnic in the boot of the car and told Sahar I wanted to go for a bushwalk down the coast. I knew of a nice viewpoint overlooking one of the world's renowned surf spots, and decided to take her there.

On the drive down, Sahar suspected nothing out of the ordinary. We arrived, parked the car, and made a start on our walk to Shipstern Bluff. Sahar isn't a fan of bushwalking and complained all the way up to the lookout. It is by no means a difficult walk, but for the whole 45 minutes she did a fair amount of whinging.

"Mitch! Are we there yet? I'm so tired!" she moaned. "This was a bad idea ... Is the lookout in sight yet?"

I could feel the engagement ring in my pocket, and I was anxious to get to the lookout so I could finally ask the question. I knew if we turned around her complaining would stop. So I kept reassuring her that we were almost there and that the view from the top would be worth it. Finally we reached the lookout and Sahar's face lit up. Out came her mobile and selfie stick, and so began the taking of a thousand selfies, couple shots, and even more of the most spectacular cliff-top views.

We enjoyed the sea breeze and view for about 20 minutes. The whole time I was just waiting for my moment to take out the ring and pop the question. I could feel my anxiety building when, each time she pulled me close for a selfie, I was sure she was going to feel the little ring box stowed away in my jacket.

Sahar had finally had enough and began walking back to the car.

"Let's go!" she said.

I knew this was my time to act, now or never.

"Come over here," I said. I hadn't moved from the lookout. She returned, a little disgruntled, and stood in front of me thinking that I wanted to get one last photo.

"Are you OK, Mitch? You look a little pale ..." she said.

I reached for the ring box, making sure it was accessible in my jacket, and pulled out the card I wanted to give her. I could feel myself breaking out in a sweat. I was about to propose to the love of my life. My hands were clammy as I handed Sahar the card and asked her to read it.

Beautiful, funny, amazing and smart.

These values you have, they rule my heart.

We have jumped some hurdles, with many to follow, but without your love, my heart would be hollow.

I'm sure you know that I'll do all I can, to keep you happy and be your man.

I see you, I stop, I think from a far, we found love, right where we are.

This ring is a symbol of my love for life, Sahar Mohamad will you be my wife?

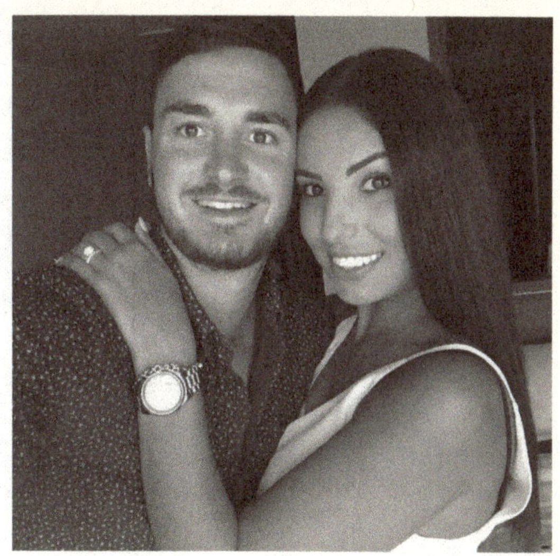

Sahar and I were fortunate enough to honeymoon in the Maldives in 2016.

As she read out the final line I pulled out the ring box and got down on one knee.

"Sahar, will you marry me?" I asked.

She was over the moon.

"Yes, yes, yes!" she cried.

It is fair to say that the 45 minute walk back to the car was much more enjoyable for both of us and there were no more complaints. We stopped along the way to ring our closest family and friends to let them know our happy news. I had packed a picnic in the boot of the car but we were way too excited to enjoy it. Instead, we took it straight down to Dad and Koula's house and called some of our best friends to come over and celebrate with us.

We were married just over a year later, on February 13, 2016. It was a traditional Arab wedding (with a touch of Aussie) filled with 280 guests. It was the most amazing day of my life.

Wedding days are a huge day for everyone. But I can't help but feel how ours was a bigger deal than for

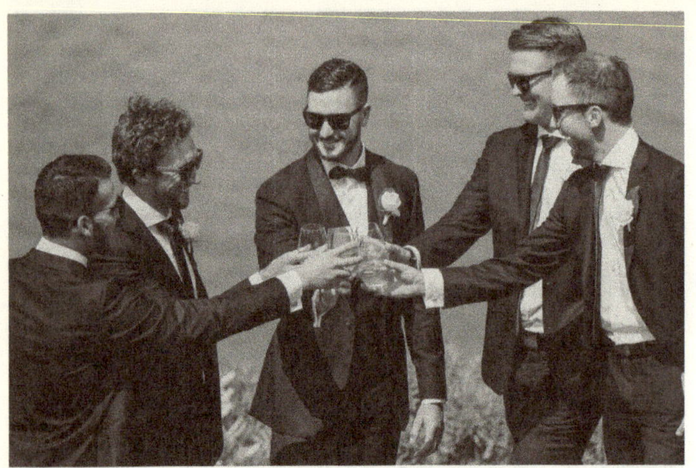

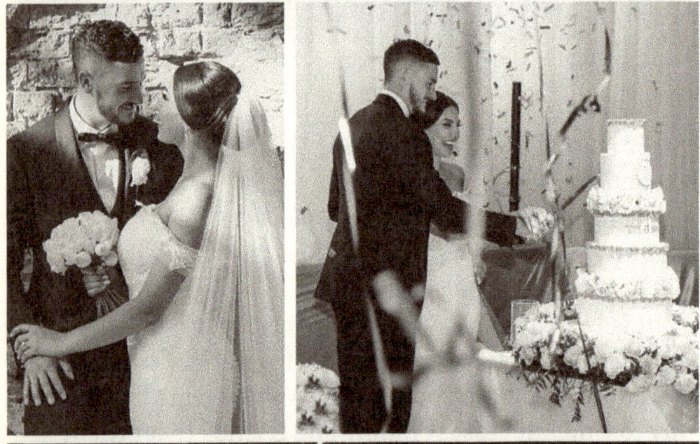

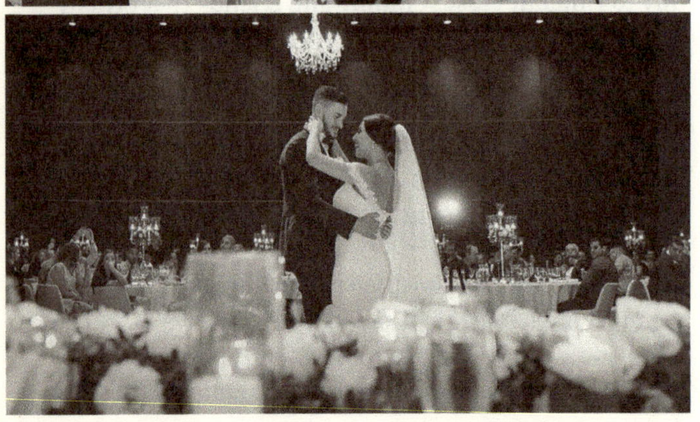

most. We had overcome all the hurdles that we'd been faced with and our dreams had finally come true.

Sahar and I walked into the reception in the evening, after a traditional Arab ceremony at home. The room was filled with people wearing the biggest smiles, clapping in time with the music and drums, and as we entered, we were introduced as husband and wife. Sahar is a big flower person. I can see how they light her up. Flowers were in bloom all over the room: all along the front of the bridal table, the cake table, and in the centre of each guest table. A large chandelier was decorated with two breathtaking halos of flowers. A five-tier white chocolate mud cake was inscribed with our wedding date in Roman numerals – the room looked amazing!

At the side of the stage was further proof, as if it was needed, of Sahar's incredible thoughtfulness. It's one of the reasons I love her so much. She had organised a small table and placed a photo of Ty on it, one that we all loved, down on one knee blowing a kiss to the camera. Next to it was another frame with the words,

We know you'd be here today if heaven wasn't so far away.

Ty, Nan and Pop were all missing from our wedding day, the three people I most wanted to be there. In the lead up to the wedding, I had been struggling with conflicting emotions – feeling so happy about this next chapter of my life, yet feeling so sad and guilty that I was moving on without Ty. Dad felt it the most. Could we celebrate so soon after our loss?

Opposite: Our wedding – a day that we will treasure forever, with 280 people joining us as we celebrated into the night.

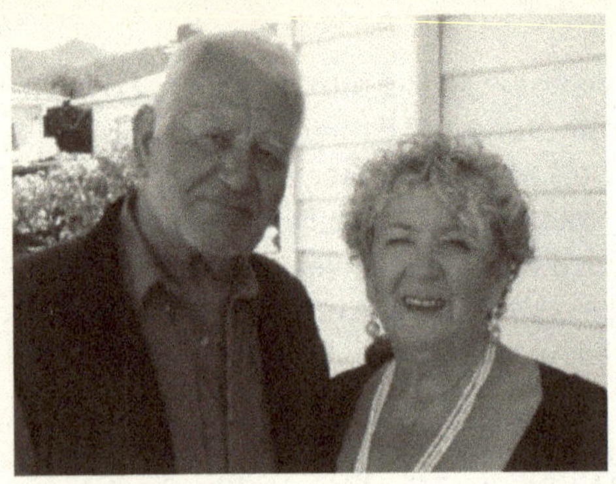

The older I get, the more I find that I miss the love and support I always received from my late Nan and Pop.

But after seeing Sahar's gesture, I felt at ease. I knew I could still love and honour Ty while being happy for myself. Ty would have wanted that. Sahar's touch was all class and I owe her a lot for thinking of it when she had so much else on her mind.

I HOPE I WILL always make Sahar laugh and feel safe and supported. Every day when I wake up I am reminded of how beautiful she is, and how lucky I am to call her my wife. I respect her loyalty to family, work, and friends, and her enthusiasm for life. She gives her all in everything while bringing out the best in me. I get so much out of caring for her, delighting her and being romantic. I like to surprise her with trips away, and have flowers waiting for her when she gets home after a bad day at work. I'll always try to make the most out of any situation we're in.

Sahar calls me her tall, handsome, funny, loving man and in her words, "when she counts her blessings, she counts me twice." She has seen me go through everything, so many dark days, and still wanted to spend forever with me. In a way I feel I have earned her love. I know it was hard for her and that at one stage she couldn't imagine ever getting to the point of telling her family about us. Eventually she could see the light at the end of the tunnel and I am so happy she decided to spend her life with me.

Losing Ty brought us closer than ever. We both learned to be more grateful, to appreciate the small things in life and look out for those around us that little bit more. I love how Sahar can see me so passionate about my job. She will never hear "I don't want to go to work today" from me any more. The way I see it, every day I get a chance open people's eyes and keep people from making the mistakes I did. To potentially save a life.

We have built a beautiful home together and rarely a week goes by without Sahar's Mum Najla telling me how much she loves me. Their family is huge and we visit them two or three times a week. It is fantastic being a part of such an amazing community of loving and caring people.

I now have a bond with Sahar's three younger brothers that will never be broken. I lost that older-brother relationship when I lost Ty. It meant so much, and now I feel like I've found it again. The three boys, Hassan, Sleiman and Haidar, are so important to me. I like to think I am a role model for them, just like I was to Tig. They don't realise the joy they have brought to my life by simply being kind, fun, and loving boys to me.

I am forever in debt for the support Sahar has shown me throughout this tragic roller coaster. Without her, I have no idea where I would be. The fact that she met Ty, that she connected with him, and can keep his memory alive with me warms my heart every day. And I could not do what I do without Sahar – she teaches me every day to be more open with my emotions and lean on people instead of hiding away.

Dad has been with Koula for the past eight years and they married recently in Hobart. I love getting up

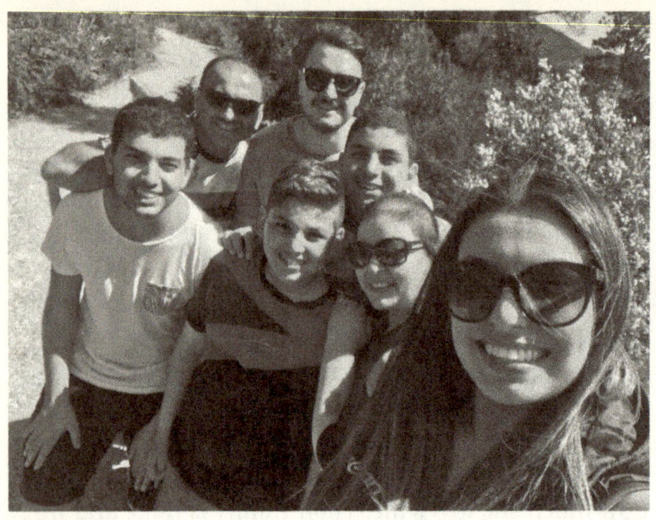

Day trips with my in-laws are an absolute favourite these days. My father-in-law Saad, mother-in-law Najla, and brothers-in-law Hassan, Sleiman and Haidar.

and speaking in front of people now, so they asked me to be their MC. Koula brings a light into Dad's world that is amazing to see. She is caring, funny, loving, and most importantly, she adores Dad. Seeing how in love they are is at times sickening, but I sleep well knowing Dad is happy.

I am still close to Koula's two children, Emmanuel and Athina. Emmanuel was one of the groomsmen at our wedding. He lives in Melbourne now with his girlfriend, playing soccer and doing his best to fit into the Melbourne fashion scene. I am lucky Emmanuel and I get on like we do and I am proud to call him my brother.

Mum married Glenn seven years ago. They separated for about a year, but fortunately now have found their way back together. I know that the break had a lot to do with Ty's passing, with how much it changed them both. Mum, mostly.

It took me a long time to understand how Mum was feeling. Her grief was, and is, intense. It still affects her in unexpected ways, six years on. No matter where she is or what she's doing – at work, driving, cooking – her mind wanders. She'll think of a memory, or just see somebody who looks like Ty, and the reality will overwhelm her again without warning.

Mum wonders what Ty would look like now, what he'd be doing with his life. She still thinks of things she needs to tell him. She's withdrawn a lot and needs to be on her own. She doesn't want to answer her phone or visit friends any more. Sometimes if you visit her she'll pretend she's not home. Mum's had three jobs since losing Ty, but now she finally has a job she loves at Hobart airport. She says she tries so hard to conceal her emptiness at work, but she still has to leave the floor sometimes because she just can't stop crying.

My Dad Dale and his amazing wife (my step-mum) Koula. They have been huge supports on both Tour de Tig events (running from Burnie to Hobart).

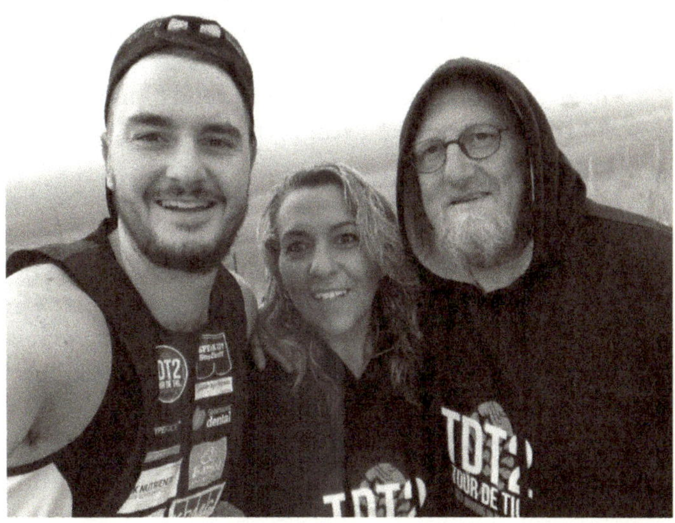

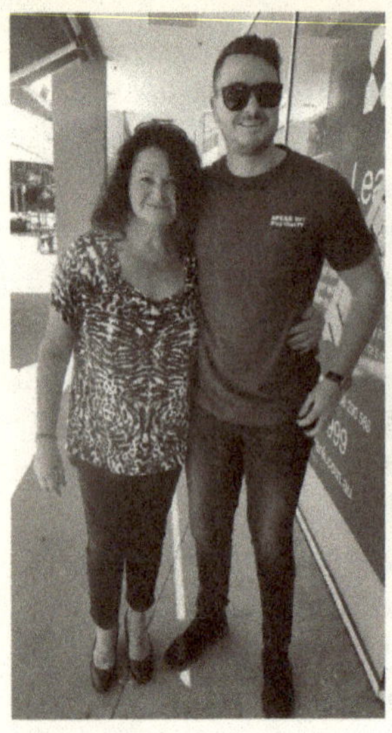

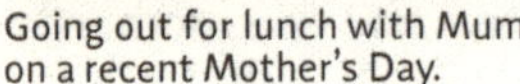

Going out for lunch with Mum on a recent Mother's Day.

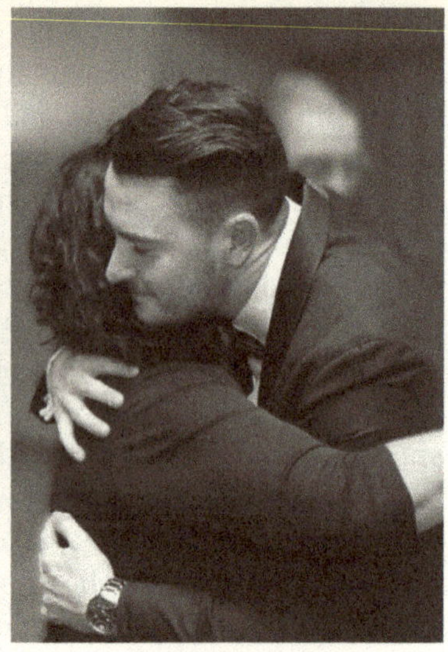

Embracing Mum at the recent Stay ChatTY Gala Ball held in Hobart.

I had coffee with Mum recently, and out of nowhere, she started crying. There was no obvious reason, we hadn't even been talking about Ty. It was really sad to see. In a way, she will forever be broken.

"I'm getting there," she told me. "I've begun to have positive moments, finally. I'm teaching myself to be happy again. I want to make Ty proud of me every day. I guess that's the one thought that keeps me going."

Mum loved Ty more than anything and wishes every day she could hold him and tell him things will be OK. She is proud of what I'm doing now. She says there's nothing more important than reaching out for help when we need it. And she wants everyone to learn to do that together, so fewer people have to bear the sadness that our family now carries.

CHAPTER 10
Discovering my purpose

SIX MONTHS after losing Ty, I came up with the idea of a car bumper sticker that could pay tribute to him. I was playing around with words with 'Ty' in them to get a slogan or saying that suited, and that's where SPEAK UP! Stay ChatTY first started. I didn't start it as a suicide awareness campaign. I just thought the sticker would help us through this dark time – mainly I wanted us as a family, our friends, to stick them on our cars – to have a laugh and a smile whenever we saw them. I wanted people to see the sticker and be reminded to check in with their loved ones and ask how they were.

I went to a signwriter friend and explained the sticker idea. We talked about the things that reminded us of Ty – what made us laugh. Ty always wore footy shorts. It was his thing. On the field, at home, even out to dinner or to barbecues, Ty was constantly in his footy shorts, usually (and uncomfortably for us), without undies. So when the idea of a sticker featuring Ty's shorts came about, I loved it. A good friend of mine arranged to have them printed, then Koula and I shared them on Facebook, charging $1 to send them out. We wanted to donate the money to an organisation we had heard about, Albie House, an organisation trying to set up supportive

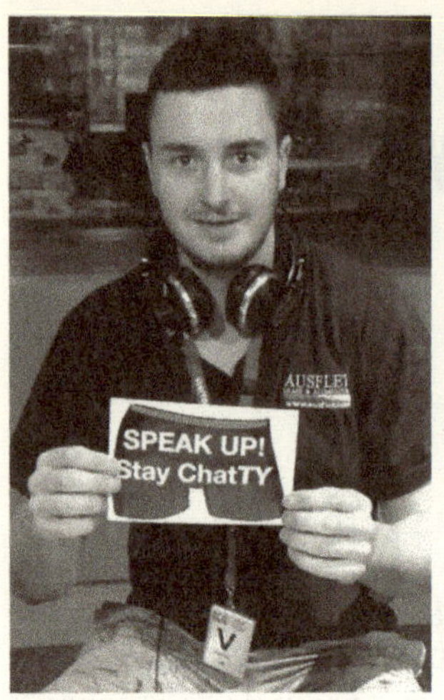

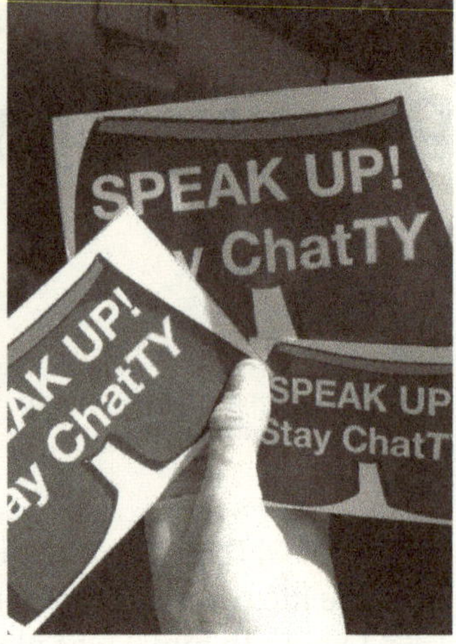

My first ever radio interview with ABC's Ryk Goddard. After creating the Stay ChatTY sticker to lift our spirits, I soon realised that change needed to be made in the way we as humans view mental health.

accommodation for people experiencing suicidal thoughts.

It wasn't long before Koula and I were flat out keeping up with posting out orders. Stay ChatTY was fast becoming a campaign that lots of people in the south of Tasmania were learning about. The stickers and my Facebook page were really hitting home for a lot of families.

I was still working as a glazier and trying to fit back into life as best I could. But this campaign was starting to take over in all the right ways. I began to see a future in this silly little idea, and nothing was going to stop me from turning it something more.

People described the campaign as a great initiative, and one that could really benefit Tasmania. Our state had, and still has, the second highest rate of suicide in Australia. This type of work was needed to bring suicide out of the shadows, and I felt that building this initiative could make a real difference. We might finally find a positive in our family's tragedy.

Our Stay ChatTY shorts is now one of the most prominent car stickers you see in Tasmania. To date, over 33,000 have been distributed not only in Tasmania, but across the country. You spot them on cars, utes and buses. They pop up on school lockers, laptops, public toilets ... all sorts of weird and wonderful places! I'm humbled when someone tells me how often they see the sticker on their travels.

The idea of that sticker changed my life. It allowed me to leave my work as a glazier and spread a positive message of hope, raising awareness of suicide and encouraging people to seek help if they need it.

AFTER SELLING STICKERS for a few months, things started to snowball in the best possible way. Momentum was building and the buzz had started to spread to families around Hobart. I ordered wristbands, seeing them as another good option for people to wear, and set up a Facebook page. To my amazement the page gathered more than 3,000 'Likes' in the first two days, and now sits at over 24,000.

While sharing my thoughts and feelings around the loss of my little brother, I also shared beyondblue and Lifeline tips on how to spot the signs and start a conversation. In a short amount of time I was starting to be seen as an advocate for suicide prevention. Social media was turning us into something people needed – a very real avenue focussed on mental health. Many people said Tasmania hadn't seen anything like this before.

There were and continue to be amazing mental health organisations in Tasmania. But I think our success was because we were a local story. Rather than being founded in another state or country, our charity was run by a local guy looking to make a difference out of a tragedy he and his family had had experienced. I think our effort resonated with people because it had happened in their own backyard.

Stay ChatTY was breaking down barriers by rallying the community around the importance of talking about mental health and suicide.

OVER THE NEXT few months my life was crazy. It was a strange feeling. Here I was, at 25, burdened by so much sadness, but at the same time finding life exciting, energised by the prospect of creating something that could make a difference and be a positive influence on others. While running around dropping off wristbands and staying up late with Koula mailing out stickers, I was on a high. Then I'd get home after a long day and the real reason why I was so busy would hit me like a tonne of bricks. I would break down.

There are so many highlights I sit back and reflect on. One, when my good mate, AFL star Jack Riewoldt, offered to show off the logo on the AFL Footy Show. Jack was a year behind me through high school. Whilst I was aware of his presence we didn't have a lot to do with each other back then. We really met over fooy. We played on the same team then started college together in 2015, and our group of mates all merged at that time.

After Jack asked about spruiking the logo on the AFL Footy Show, I had the logo blown up to A3 size and express mailed it to Melbourne in time for the show.

I knew what I was involved in was special, but at this stage it was very unclear to me what I wanted to do with the awareness I was raising. All I knew was that I wanted as many people as possible to see our logo and to know that it stood for the power of a conversation. There was no doubt Jack's support was going to assist with that.

Before the show, I posted on my Facebook page, "Make sure everyone watches the Footy Show tonight, our boy Jacky Riewoldt is going to mention Stay ChatTY". So many people left comments saying they would be tuning in and there was a real buzz in our household in anticipation.

That night I sat by myself in my room to watch the show. It was an agonising wait and it wasn't until the last two minutes of the show that Jack brought out the A3 logo I'd sent him. He sat there with our logo on the desk and began speaking about the work I was doing. He told viewers he had seen the devastation that this had caused, that he fully supported our work, and encouraged people to visit the Facebook page and show support.

I sat on the edge of my bed crying.

"That was all right, hey mate?" Dad yelled out from the top of the stairs.

"Yeah awesome," I said, wiping away tears, hoping Dad wouldn't come down to my room. Dad had seen me shed plenty of tears over the last few months, and it wouldn't have mattered if he saw me crying again.

AFL star Jack Riewoldt is a great friend. His ongoing support and initiatives at early stages of Stay ChatTY have helped build the profile of our organisation.

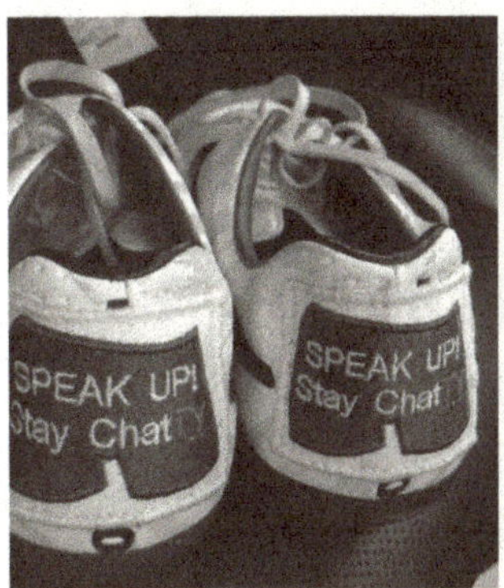

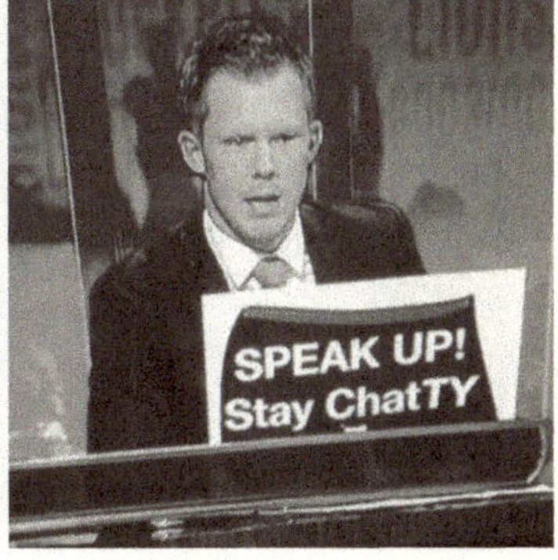

But at that moment I just didn't want to explain why the tears were there.

Seeing Jack on the AFL Footy Show paying tribute to Ty and pledging support to suicide prevention really was a big moment. I knew our efforts were going to lead to a big future. I guess it was my first realisation that the work I had been doing might lead to something bigger than just a small campaign in Hobart – and I think this was the source of my tears.

AS TIME PASSED, I decided that a statewide event would lift the profile of the campaign to a new level. After a few phone calls to my mates, and chats with Dad at home around the kitchen table, I drummed up the idea of "Tour de Tig". Myself and six of my mates were going to run from Burnie to Hobart (360 km) in just four and a half days. Planning got under way and it dominated my life for the next few months.

We ran the Tour de Tig in late February 2014, just over a year after Ty's passing. Along the way we stopped in towns for fundraisers, and met and cried with so many people. Thanks to an amazing support crew, we battled the bitumen for five days. The media

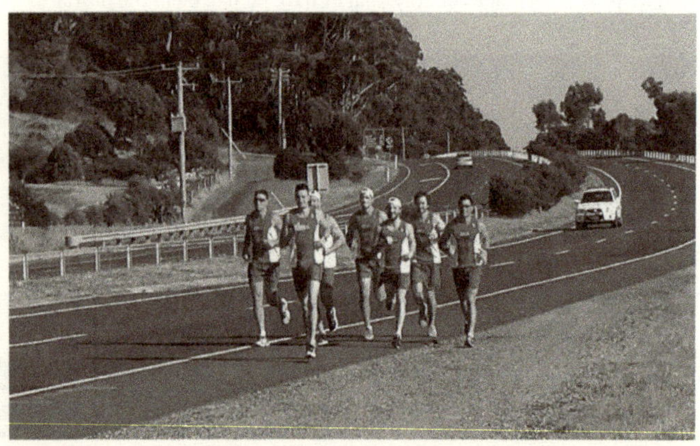

got behind us, from newspapers to news crews, and we lit up social media as much as we could, sharing the journey and battles we were putting ourselves through.

For the final two kilometres we decided to group up and run on to Hobart's regatta ground in front of more than 150 friends and family. I ran the final leg, detouring off into the cemetery where Ty now lies. I knew this would be a really touching moment for all of us.

I ran into the cemetery that day with all the boys and support crew behind me. I had my favourite song, "Mirrors" by Justin Timberlake, playing through my headphones, reminding me of Ty. I knew that song would make me emotional. In a way I was doing my best to be emotional. I just wanted to get to Ty and let it all out. All the planning, all the organising, the hard work that had gone into this event had taken its toll.

When I finally reached his grave facing out over the Derwent River, I was bawling my eyes out. I was exhausted and overcome with emotion when the rest of the support crew stepped out of their cars. We all hugged and cried around Ty's gravesite, and I look

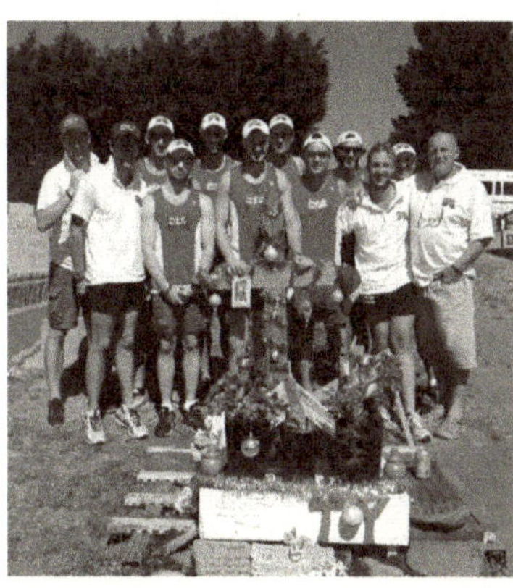

Opposite: In January 2014 Tour de Tig 1 saw me and six mates (Ben Fagan, Tim Orchard, Nick Paine, Rohan Swan, Sam Iles and Ben Langford) run 360 kilometres in four and a half days to help launch Stay ChatTY across Tasmania.

Left: Running in to the cemetery to see Ty on the final day of the tour was one of the most emotional moments in my life — elation mixed with the realisation of why we had put ourselves through this challenge was an overwhelming feeling.

back on that moment with so much pride. We had all battled soreness, tiredness, and sleeping in a different bed every night for a week, but we had kept going. This was a tribute to our mate, but our underlying message was to make everyone aware of the pain suicide causes those left behind. We wanted anyone struggling in silence to know that we saw them, we recognised they were suffering and wanted them to reach out. And we wanted to remind everyone around them of the importance of listening, and asking those tough questions.

Tour de Tig 1 raised more than $20,000. The lead up, the week, and the days that followed will forever be a highlight in my life. I was, and continue to be, conscious of the fact that events don't come together thanks to one person. So many people and businesses contributed to TDT1, and I wanted to ensure that everyone who contributed came together at the end and were thanked as a group. I organised a function room in Hobart's Salamanca for more than 120 supporters to celebrate and recognise the achievements of that week. I was able to thank everyone without breaking down, but as soon as I opened up about Ty, I lost control.

AFTER THE RUN, life returned to normal in many ways. I was no longer juggling 38 hours of work as a glazier and organising an event. Life had quietened down. But I felt lost and hated not feeling busy as hell. More than that, it made me realise how much I wanted to keep going with what we'd started.

Over the subsequent weeks, I did some reflecting. I went over the run in my mind, especially the amount of support we were shown, purely because so many people had been touched by suicide. People had pulled up alongside us to donate money, they had messaged

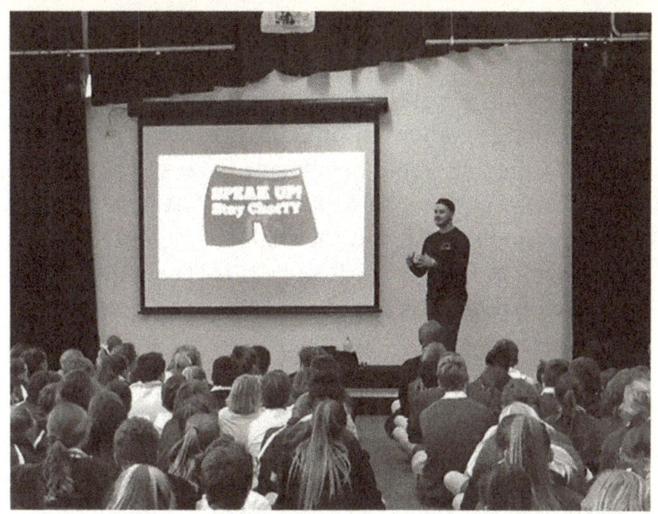

I had never done much public speaking. But the feedback that my presentation was really engaging gave me the confidence to go forward. Speaking with school groups (such as Mackillop College, shown here in 2016) was and is a very rewarding experience.

our Facebook page opening up about their own experiences, and contacted us to tell us how proud they were. They encouraged us to keep Stay ChatTY going, telling us we would save lives.

I decided to set up Stay ChatTY as a registered not-for-profit organisation. To do this, I received a lot of help from friends of friends, a lawyer and an accountant, who knew this line of work and wanted to dedicate their time to help me achieve my goals.

After being invited to some local footy clubs and schools to talk about Stay ChatTY, I started to understand what it was that I wanted to actually do with the organisation. My calling was to share my story. I hoped that sharing my own heartache and tears, the devastation that suicide had caused my family, would help others talk more openly about the issue. I wanted to help people see they do not have to struggle alone.

I knew I couldn't change the world overnight or, like Superman, single-handedly save people's lives. But I wished someone had told me my own story before Ty died. It would have made me see that mental health issues and suicide are a reality. That they are prevalent and painful, but they can be prevented and treated. It would have made me realise the importance of breaking down the stigma and checking in with the ones you love.

NOW, when I meet people bereaved by suicide, I feel their pain. I have a respect for their strength, and a connection, knowing we share the same emotional devastation. We share the same story. We know how deep the pain runs. We know that despite it, we still get up every day, have a shower and get dressed – as hard as it is. We know the dark hole we've been in. I recognise their journey, their grief, their Facebook statuses. I share the what-ifs, the guilt. I share the look that questions whether there was something we could have done for our loved ones, and the fear of admitting it to ourselves.

That's why we need to challenge our ignorance and become more aware of mental health issues and suicide. So that people can find other options than suicide, and families and communities don't have to live with this pain.

Since Ty's death, I have heard of several young men around Ty's age who have taken their own lives. These boys would have heard messages about mental health. I know they would have heard about suicide prevention. But they're still dying by suicide.

That's why mental health promotion and suicide prevention are everyone's business. We need to raise awareness, but we also need to normalise feelings, teach people how to express them, and teach the community to support these conversations. We need to stop the stigma and make it OK for people, especially young people, to feel and to cry and to lean on each other.

One in five people will experience a mental health issue in their lifetime, which means if you know more than five people, chances are one of them is struggling. They are not stupid. They are not different. They are not ungrateful or dramatic. They are going through something they need help with. And we as a community need to be ready and willing to give that help.

My good mate Ben Langford was a huge support through out the initial journey of getting Stay ChatTY off the ground.

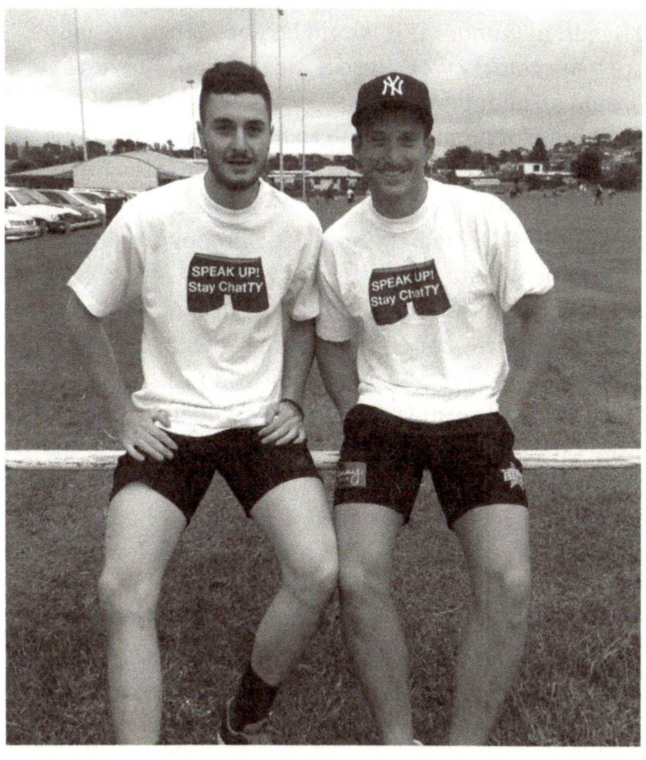

CHAPTER 11

Tradie turned public speaker

IN JUNE 2014, momentum was big around SPEAK UP! Stay ChatTY. I was taking a lot of time off work as a glazier to attend mental health events and give presentations to community groups across Tasmania. I began to wonder if it would be possible to actually turn my charity work into a fulltime job, and how I would go about doing this.

I was fortunate enough to meet Mat Rowell and Michael Kelly, CEO and COO of Relationships Australia Tasmania, after their organisation made a donation to Tour de Tig 1 to help fund accommodation for everyone who took part.

Over some weeks, I shared my dreams and ideas with them over coffee. I began to see Relationships Australia Tasmania as an organisation that might take me on and allow me to pursue my wild idea to take Stay ChatTY to the next level.

My first interview was at their office on a Friday afternoon. I had just finished work, and rolled in wearing my silicone-covered tradie polo, shorts and boots — not quite what they were expecting. I told them of my desire to create a schools program, to share my story in sporting clubs, and to travel the state encouraging conversations at workplaces about mental health. Much to my excitement, they decided to employ me three days a week and bring Stay ChatTY under the RA Tas wing to see how it all would go.

I had their complete backing: a desk, office, and access to mental health counsellors who could attend speaking engagements with me. They would put me through mental health training and speaking courses. They offered me whatever I needed to strengthen and improve my work. Stay ChatTY was now auspiced by an organisation that could take it to the next level, and I hoped I could reach many more lives across Tasmania.

I will always remember the exciting conversations I had with Sahar about this next stage, stoked to tell her about the organisation that was prepared to back me. It felt incredible to think this could actually be my job. Friends and family were so supportive and encouraged me to grab this opportunity with both hands.

The next challenge was to tell my glazing team. I knew this was going to be tough. Scott had sensed for a while that this was the direction I hoped to take. I continued to work as a glazier for two days a week, with three days at RA Tas, but it wasn't sustainable. Presentation requests, invites to attend stalls, requests to partner with Stay ChatTY — the invitations grew over the next couple of months. I told Mat and Michael that I was finding it impossible to handle everything in just three days. Could we make it five? Again, to my delight, they agreed.

In August 2018, I ticked over four years as an employee of Relationships Australia Tasmania. What a whirlwind it has been.

The partnership between Stay ChatTY and Relationships Australia has never been stronger. We have full-time staff working on our Schools Program, our Sports Program, running day-to-day operations and finding new ways to grow. We travel to schools across the state talking about mental health, help-seeking and

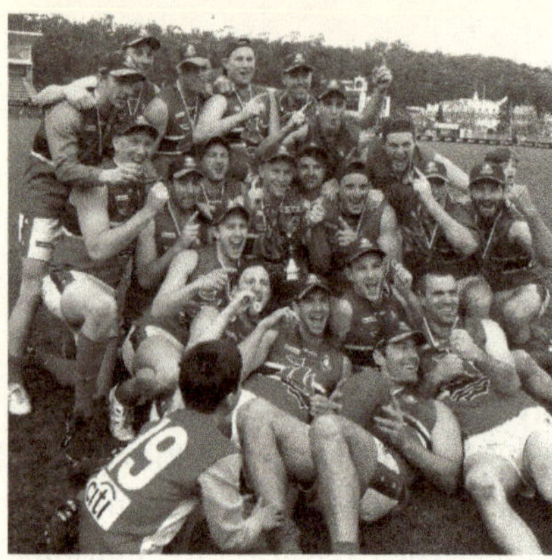

Left: Winning a premiership in 2011 with so many good mates at the OHA Football Club was definitely the biggest highlight of my sporting career. That season we went 20-0.

Opposite: Speaking to the 600 strong crowd at the first Stay ChatTY Gala Ball was a moving experience and my biggest crowd to date.

supporting our friends. We work with sports clubs to raise awareness about mental health, resilience and performance, and help them run sporting rounds where they wear our logo proudly. I continue to share my story with the many passionate and empathetic people in Tasmania who want to make a difference.

We have partnered with some major Tasmanian organisations like Fairbrother, Banjos, St Lukes Health, DJ Motors, NAB, Zest Advertising and many more. We host an annual golf day, and the biggest event we hold is our Annual Gala Ball, which celebrates everyone who has supported us over the year and raises funds for our work.

I still feel overwhelmed with gratitude at the amount of support and encouragement we receive from our community. We wouldn't be here today without it, and it shows me that this cause is worth pursuing.

I can't explain what it means to me to finally be doing something that gives my life meaning. Thinking back about the emotion and drive I had to make something out of Stay ChatTY makes me so proud of who I've become. If there was such a thing as destiny, I was convinced this was mine.

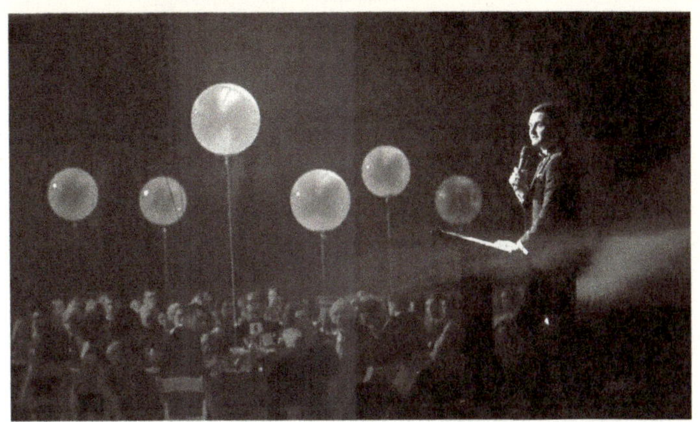

AS THE CHARITY grows in leaps and bounds, one of the most commonly asked questions I get is, "How do you know if you are making a difference?" I don't know the statistics on how many people's lives we may have changed by telling Ty's story — that we will never know.

Early on, I received a message from a follower on our Facebook page. It was one of the first moving pieces of feedback I had gotten, and gave me that reassurance that what I was doing was right:

Mitch, how are you going mate? I don't know you, nor do you know me, but I have decided to write you a message anyway. Hopefully it will brighten your day and give you an extra boost of confidence that what you are doing is amazing.

From my mid-teens, I struggled with severe anxiety and depression. They weren't linked, my anxiety is my anxiety and my depression is my depression. Getting into party drugs in my late teens and early twenties sent me into a downward spiral.

I grew up in a loving, normal family, and so I felt ungrateful about how negative I was feeling. Like I didn't realise how lucky I was. So I didn't talk about what I was going through. I hid behind the smiles and the laughs.

I got to the point where some days I was scared to be alone when I was messed up on drugs or drunk. I would think about killing myself. I would consider it. The thought for some reason sometimes made me happy. Like I was happy to leave it all behind.

One night a few years ago, I had just got back from town. I was pretty messed up and I decided to message the SPEAK UP! Stay ChatTY page. I received a reply which asked if I was okay. They gave me some numbers to reach out to. After a week or so I worked up the courage to call and make an appointment with a counsellor. It was hard to walk in that door and admit to myself that I was not okay. Speaking to her changed everything. I told my family, my close friends. I moved back home. I cleaned up my life. I stopped hanging out with people that brought me down, and instead hung out with people that lifted me up. I still struggle some days as we all do, but now I try to be open with how I'm feeling.

In the end I left Tassie to leave old memories behind and make some new ones. Tassie will always be my home and I know I'll be back when I'm ready.

This all started with you brother. It started with your page. I'd seen the logo around and it was my first and possibly last attempt at calling out for help. I'm sure this is one story of many that you've heard. I just want you to know that quite possibly, your page saved my life.

Now I'm excited about life. I wake up every day looking forward to my adventure. Sure some days I'm not okay, but I'll never forget that it's okay to speak up and that it's okay to not be okay.

You're a legend. Thank you.

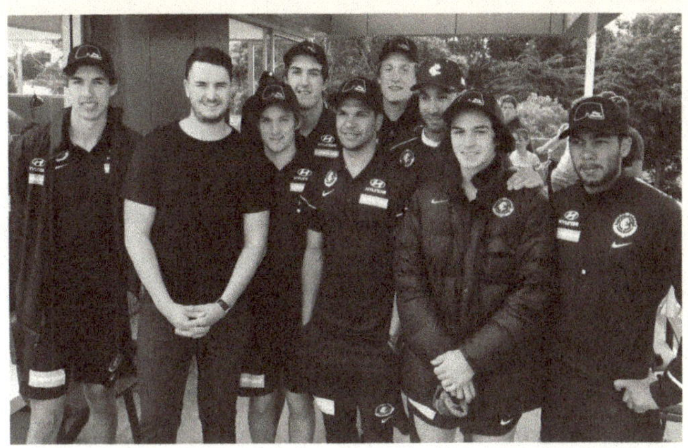

As a Carlton Football Club fan, being asked by my former coach Brendan Bolton to address the first and second year players in early 2017 was a tremendous honour.

I've stopped counting the messages I get from kids who tell me that thanks to hearing my talk, they went to see a counsellor. All I know is, with Ty in my sights, I have that drive and that fire to do the best I can for our community.

I CONFESS THAT sometimes I'm numb when talking about losing Ty. I share my story so much now it becomes habit, and in some ways, I need to distance myself from that pain in order to share. A self-preservation thing, I guess. But I can't fall into the trap of lessening or sanitising my grief. People connect and change through the power of emotions, and I can't lose the strength of that connection.

In the early days I was smashing out presentations, doing as many as I could to get the message out and the charity up and running. One day I found myself sobbing at work about how much it was getting to me, how I just couldn't turn my brain off. I was dwelling too much on Ty, thinking about painful memories and getting stuck in those never-ending loops. It was bringing me down and I was beginning to burn out.

Now, with the help of the RA Tas and my own team, we set standards and rules around my work so I don't burn out. I know now that I need to put limits on my work to keep myself safe. I need to take care of myself so I can continue to share my story, share my grief in a constructive way that engages and connects. I can't lose that impact.

THE SPEAKING SIDE of my role hasn't always been easy. I faced so many challenges in making that transition from tradie to public speaker. Fear, lack of confidence, lack of credibility. In the beginning my delivery was poor, and I was unfamiliar with some of the necessary messages I needed to share. Above all, I needed the respect and confidences of my audiences if I were to have an impact. Who was Mitch McPherson? What were these silly shorts stickers?

When I officially began working with RA Tas, one of my first invitations was to present to an organisation's training day for 60 staff. They had heard about Stay ChatTY, and felt that a focus on mental health and suicide prevention was something their workplace really needed.

I travelled to the site, about 40 minutes out of Hobart, arriving half an hour early as planned. I signed in, made my way to the presentation area and sat down in the kitchen until a woman came to greet me.

"Welcome Mitch, thank you so much for coming," she said. "You are rather early, so take a seat, help yourself to tea or coffee, and I will come and grab you when it's time to present."

I started to panic. Pre-presentation anxiety was setting in. I had only done a handful of talks and it always crept up on me. Normally I would have a chance to steady myself by checking the PowerPoint presentation, doing a sound check and assessing the

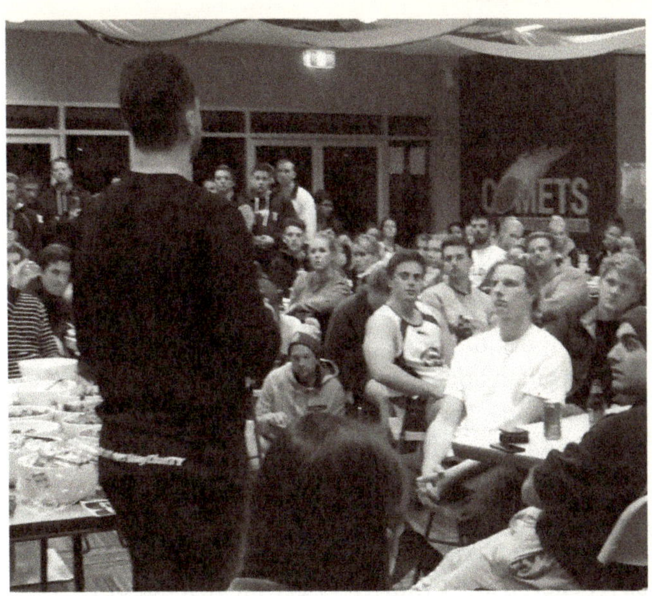

My presentations have now branched out beyond Tasmania. Here I am pictured speaking with the men's and women's teams from the Kew Football Club in Victoria.

space before the room filled with an audience. Now I realised I would have to walk in and set up with sixty people staring at me.

After four years, I feel completely relaxed standing in front of an audience and thrive in the emotion I feel when delivering my message. I've had to handle technical issues, awkward moments, people walking out or crying, and all kinds of unexpected situations. I feel at ease with whatever gets thrown at me.

But in the early days, this was far from the case. My biggest fear was forgetting the structure of my presentation. I had built up a PowerPoint with photos, videos and graphic material, essentially my guide to what I had to say. I also made small cards with everything written down, word for word, just in case. My plan was to look less at the cards so I could maintain direct eye contact with my audience.

So there I was, tucked away in the corner of a staff kitchen, frantically reading my notes, checking my PowerPoint on the laptop and sweating bullets that I was about to face my biggest audience yet. To make matters worse, the person presenting before me had the audience laughing and joking. I felt the confidence drain out of me with every passing minute and just wanted to get the whole thing over and done with.

All of a sudden the meeting room doors opened and a woman appeared. She was speaking into her mobile phone, so didn't notice me tucked in the corner. As she went by I overheard her saying, "I'll still be another hour. We've got some idiot here next to talk about suicide ..."

Already filled with self-doubt, my anxiety skyrocketed and I wanted to get the hell out of there. I lost my breath and with it my sense of perspective. I decided everyone in the room must be thinking the same. I started to text an excuse for why I had to bolt, when the doors opened again.

"We are ready for you to come in now, Mitch," the host said.

I gathered my things and followed her into the room. Head down, I started to plug in and prepare everything as quickly as I could. Thankfully, the audience was relaxed, having a break. Some were chatting, some stretching their legs. I was relieved they weren't all sitting quietly, staring at me and waiting to start.

I checked that each slide worked, made sure the sound was on, held my cards in one hand, took a sip of water, and signalled to the host that I was ready. There was no way out now.

While the host made her way to the front of the room, the audience noticed the session was about to begin and took their seats. Just at this point,

Phone Call Lady walked in and sat down in the row right in front of me. I needed to hurry up and get this done so I could get out.

I was introduced, there was applause, and finally I got under way. For the next 25 minutes, I stumbled and mumbled my way through my story. The cards slipped out of my hands and I just couldn't think clearly or focus on the job at hand. Phone Call Lady in the front row seemed to have zero interest in what I was saying, and it was impossible not to be distracted by her looking like she had better things to do.

I finished, they clapped again, and started to pack up. A number of people came up to me to say they appreciated what I had to say. Despite their words of encouragement, I left a broken man.

For so long I had been riding a high, gaining fresh employment, being told this would be amazing, and having heaps of people helping me turn the tragedy of Ty's suicide into a positive message for others.

As a tradesman, I feel I can connect well with men who are working in the trade industry. In a male-dominated work force the stigma surrounding mental health can be quite high: breaking down barriers and encouraging men to speak about their mental health is a big challenge we face.

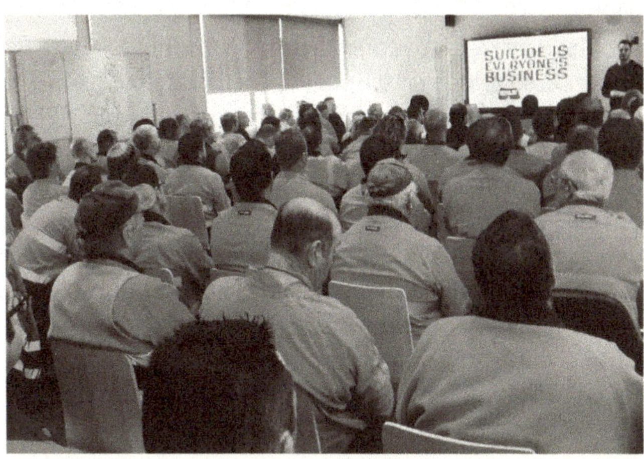

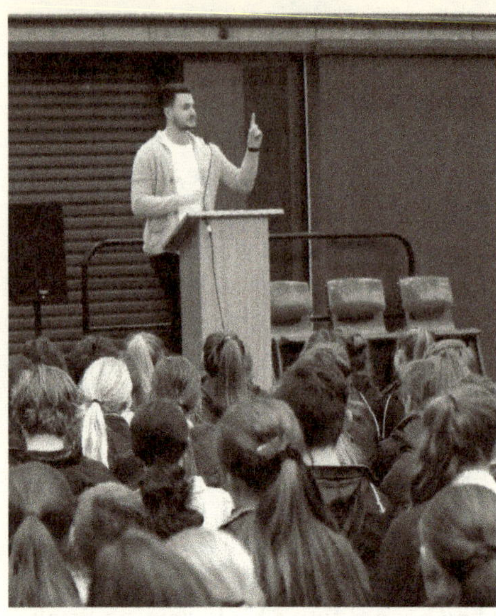

Sharing my lived experience is my passion and my purpose.

But now I had been faced with the negative side of the work I was in. I hadn't experienced a reaction like that in my journey, and it rocked me.

I couldn't shake the anxiety Phone Call Lady had provoked, so as I drove out, I rang Sahar. She tried to soothe my nerves and said, "Well, that's just how some people are".

She was right, of course. But I still couldn't understand why that woman in the front row had so little desire to hear anything to do with suicide. My immediate reaction was to assume she was completely ignorant, that she had never been touched by suicide or felt the pain of it. That was why she was so dismissive and had made me feel so uncomfortable.

I knew I disliked the woman – how rude she had been, how she had disrespected my brother, and even made me doubt my new career. But upon reflection, I started to think differently. Maybe she had been supporting someone suicidal, or had even contemplated suicide herself? If she had sat there and cried, or needed to walk out in front of her peers and colleagues, would she have been worried they would judge her or look at her differently? Perhaps she tried to cover her emotions by treating me with disdain.

Phone Call Lady taught me two major life lessons. One, never judge someone for acting differently to how you might. Take the time to find out why they are acting as they are, as the answers might surprise you.

I don't know for a fact that she was struggling or experiencing mental ill-health, but given its prevalence, she could have been. So many people act out of character to hide or cover up how they are truly feeling. Or perhaps she still held those stigmatising views about suicide, which are more often than not informed by what we see and hear around us rather than a deeply-rooted personal belief. Or maybe she had just had a shitty day. Instead, I had skipped to judgement and formed an opinion entirely based on my own feelings.

The second thing I learned is never to doubt what you believe in. It was one of my first talks and I knew I still had a lot to learn. But if I had my time again, I wouldn't have let her actions get to me. I now know that I was onto a good thing. I know that I was destined to become better at speaking, and I know that I was destined to help change this conversation around mental health and suicide.

FOUR YEARS ON, I've given over 600 talks. People say I connect, I am engaging, and I am brave. Those early days stressing through my presentation have made me who I am today.

Publicly, I have been acknowledged with community and statewide awards for the work I was doing. This was mind-blowing to me, being recognised for something that I simply felt I had to do. However, winning these awards is bittersweet. I can be standing there being told how brave I am, about the difference I am making, but I know deep down I am receiving accolades because my brother is dead.

Over the years accepting these awards has humbled me, and opened so many doors for Stay ChatTY. Some of the awards I've been given include:

- Clarence Citizen of the Year Award in 2014
- Tasmanian of the Year finalist 2014
- Southern Cross Young Achiever, Heather and Christopher Chong Community Service Award 2015
- Tasmanian Pride of Australia Medal for Community Spirit 2015
- Southern Cross Young Achiever, St Luke's Healthier Communities Award 2016
- Premier's Young Achiever of the Year Award 2016
- Red Herring Surf Communities in Action for Suicide Prevention LIFE Award 2016
- 2016 Tasmanian Community Achievement Award winner for 'Healthier Communities'
- 2017 Tasmanian Young Australian of the Year

In 2015, Sahar nominated me for Tasmanian Young Australian of the Year. I was fortunate to be named in the final three and was asked to attend the ceremony in Hobart. I didn't feel worthy to be nominated for such an award, and felt guilty because Ty wasn't around to share it with. But when I didn't win that night, I was devastated. Lots of people had wished me luck on social media, and I had started to think about the difference I could make if I did win. Missing out was tough to swallow.

In 2017 I was nominated again. I made the final four, then went on to win the bloody thing! I was, and forever will be, the 2017 Tasmanian Young Australian of the Year, easily my biggest achievement to date. Sahar and I headed to Canberra for the national awards held each year on Australia Day. We were brought together for three days with amazing young finalists from across the country.

We were treated like royalty for the whole trip, and it was an invaluable networking opportunity. We attended luncheons and dinners, were escorted everywhere, walked red carpets, met CEOs of some of Australia's biggest organisations, met the Governor General, and even visited the Prime Minister at his home.

I was sitting in Parliament House in Canberra for the awards ceremony screened live on ABC

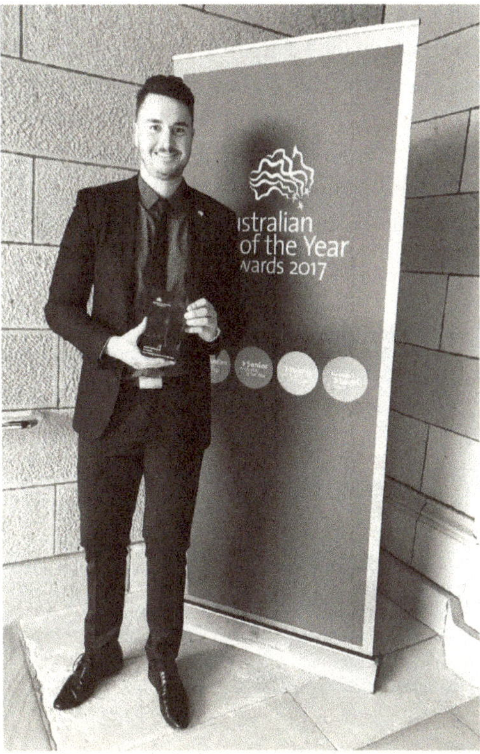

In 2017 I had the honour of being the Tasmanian Young Australian of the Year for my work in suicide prevention.

television. As they read out the winner, I remember squeezing Sahar's hand praying it would be my name. Unfortunately, I didn't win. That honour went to Paul Vasileff, owner and director of Australian fashion house Paolo Sebastian.

At the time I was upset I didn't win. It was hard not to imagine what winning could do to boost the profile of Stay ChatTY. To be able to share our story on a national scale and raise awareness for something that I really cared about would have been life-changing.

But out of the experience, I realised that while I didn't win, I have a community, a state, and a country that believes in what I'm doing and is encouraging me to keep going. And more than that, there are amazing people across the country busting their asses to make a difference to benefit other Australians. I felt so lucky to be considered part of that group.

I may win more awards, I may not. But if I do, I will stand up and say the same thing I say in every speech I have given. Winning is an amazing feeling, it makes me feel proud and it breaks my heart at the same time. But it puts mental health and suicide awareness in the spotlight, and that gives me the biggest sense of achievement of all.

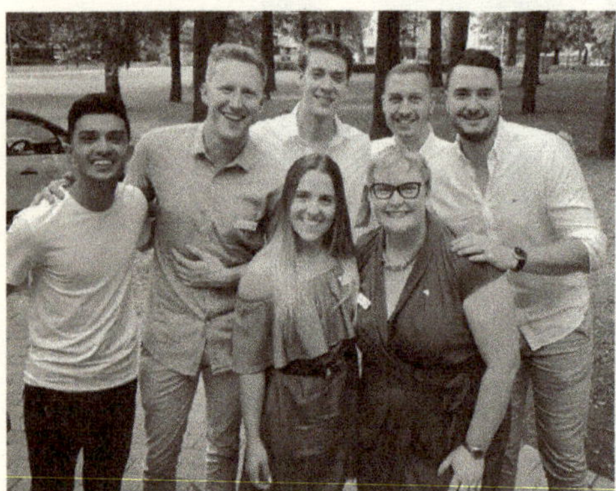

Being the Tasmanian Young Australian of the Year allowed me to travel to Canberra for the National awards on Australia Day in 2017. Here I am pictured with the other Young Australians from around the country.

CHAPTER 12

Ty's legacy

IT IS AN understatement to say that losing Ty has been life-changing. I might have stayed glazing, tucked away in the comfort of my small bubble, seeing the direction I wanted my life to take, but not having the drive to ever get there.

I used to tell Sahar about one day wanting to start my own glazing business. I thought this would help me feel accomplished and set us up financially to do the things we wanted to do. I did in fact get an ABN for Mitch's Glass. I ran with the tagline: "If your glass breaks, I've got what it takes", which of course I thought was hilarious. Now the ABN sits there unused, definitely how I prefer it.

I never set out to do what I do now and I'm amazed how many messages I receive from people looking to set up their own not-for-profit or small business. They come to me wanting to learn how we got started. I have lost track of the number of people who want to know, 'What were your first steps?' and 'What did you do to make Stay ChatTY so successful?' The only answer I can give is that I believed totally and completely in what I was working towards, and no one was going to stop me from achieving that. I meet with people wherever I can if I think my knowledge will benefit them, or help them get a leg up in whatever it is they are passionate about.

At the same time, I can't be frozen in time because of something incredibly painful that happened to me. I know I need to evolve to the next version of me.

I was far more selfish years ago. Mitch was always number one. I wasn't a bad person, but I certainly didn't have the empathy or compassion I do now. I would laugh at people's strife, brush things off as other people's problem, and focused solely on my own petty issues. Since losing Ty, I have learned I feel for people and I want to help. If someone's having a tough time I'll reach out to check in with them, make sure that everything's all right. I stand up for what I believe in, and I believe that everybody deserves respect, empathy, and someone to care.

Sahar has noticed the change in me since losing Ty. I used to hold on to grudges and be stubborn, convinced my way of seeing things was correct. But I let things go more now, and try to hang on to a positive outlook. I used to be that typical Australian man, a jock who toughed it out and never showed his feelings, lest he be ridiculed or shamed. Sahar sees me being a lot more open with my emotions, at ease talking about how I feel.

I hope that I continue to learn and grow myself in this way. I want to become more aware of the issues around me, more empathetic to people's experiences, and more inclusive of backgrounds and perspectives that are different to my own.

At work now it's not just me running the Stay ChatTY. There are many more that make the wheels turn every day, and with that brings challenges I never knew I could manage. I truly believe the one thing your team members need is to love their job. If that's not there, then the passion, the drive and the work

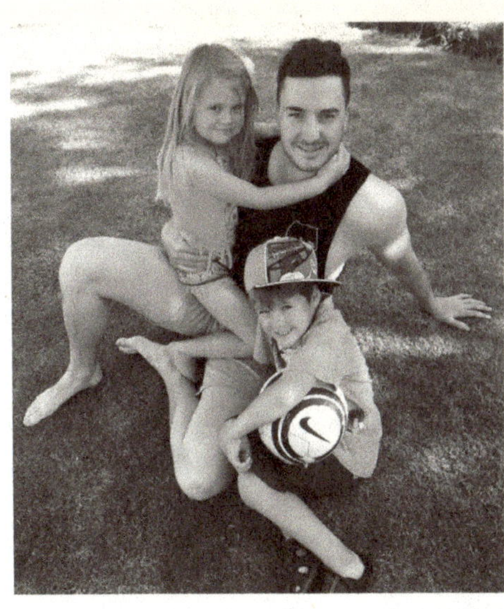

Time with my beautiful niece Ruby and nephew Brock is precious. I am so proud of my sister for raising two brilliant young kids.

ethic won't be there either. I want to know the team as best I can, to find out what inspires that love and how I can make this a job they are excited to get up every morning to do. I also want to know them better on a personal level, so that I can detect if they are having a bad day and need a chat. I try to be organised and fair, and I am certainly determined. I thank my lucky stars every day that those who work with us share the exact same aspirations for the work we do.

But I also have perspective. Losing friends and loved ones over the past five years has made me focus much more on family. I guess this has been a blessing. I still have a lot of work to do when it comes to finding time for family, but I am doing my best. We are still rebuilding after losing Ty, and our relationships haven't been the easiest to navigate since then.

I still don't feel like I'm the best uncle to my niece Ruby and nephew Brock. I find it hard to give them the time that they deserve. My sister has done a wonderful job raising them as a single parent. I don't tell her anywhere near enough, but I am so proud of her. I'm not sure I could do it on my own like she has, especially with the sadness she has faced alone. Jenna and I have had our ups-and-downs, but I would say now that we are in a good place. Having a positive relationship (even if it is mainly texts and calls) is a starting point.

If someone had asked me what my priorities were back before Ty died, I would have said my girlfriend, my mates, my family and my job. I would have said that, but I certainly wouldn't have meant it anywhere near as much as I do now. They are everything to me, my top four priorities. I know I can always do better, but at least these days I am more aware of my shortcomings, and I am trying. More importantly, I know what I need to do to keep these priorities front and centre. I communicate more, I show more compassion, I show genuine interest, and I let them know what they mean to me.

Footy was and always will be my main sport. I don't play any more due to many injuries. I had a knee reconstruction in early 2016 that made me call

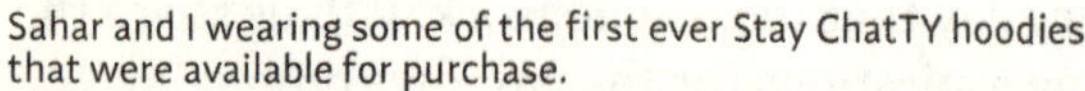

Sahar and I wearing some of the first ever Stay ChatTY hoodies that were available for purchase.

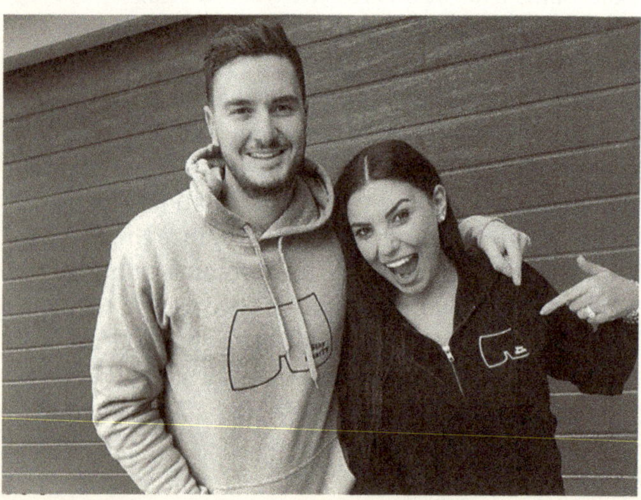

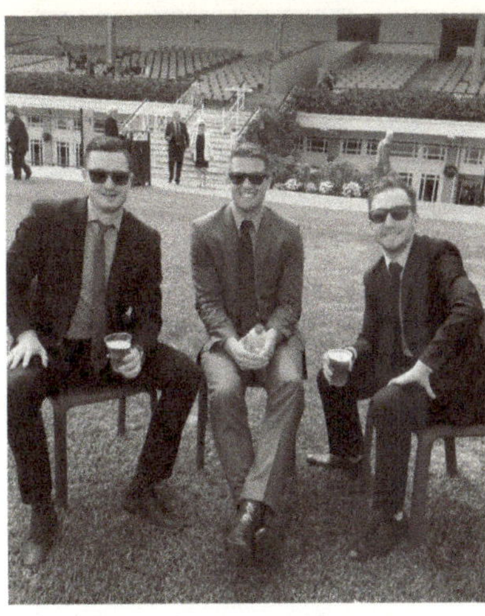

My two best mates Ben Fagan and Tim Orchard both now reside interstate. Catching up with them always brings me great joy.

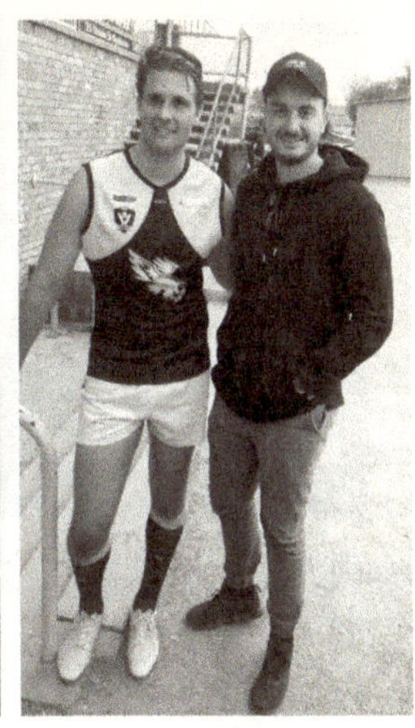

Ben played for Mansfield Football Club in Melbourne. I went to watch but sadly they lost by over 100 points …

curtains on what I tell my wife was "an illustrious career full of so many highlights …" I have gone back to my old side to do the running on game day. It's wonderful to be part of it again. Being around the lads, feeling that game day emotion that I miss so much. I would love to play again, but I'm not sure it's worth the risk of being injured.

I am confident that I am a good friend. I pride myself on asking how people are, wishing them happy birthday, making contact, catching up. I genuinely care about the people who matter most, and I try to show them rather than taking them for granted. I'm no longer selfish with my money or with my time. I realise now that the way we treat others affects us all. It can affect us greatly. These days "Take care and be kind" is one of my favourite sayings. We may not always get it right, and we may not always do it right. But being conscious of it makes a difference, and if we practice it a little bit every day, we will change for the better.

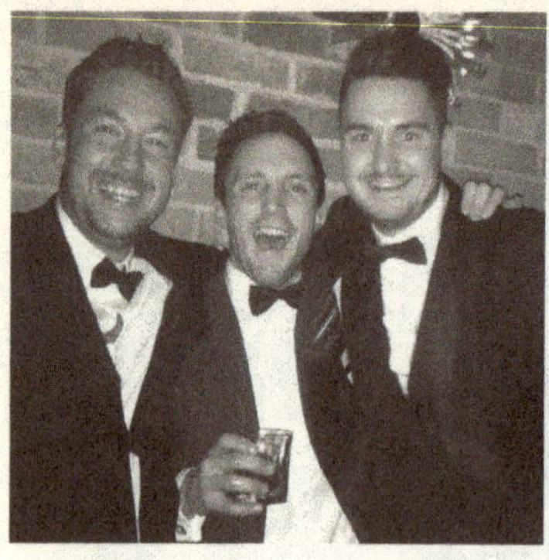

Celebrating the 2017 Stay ChatTY Ball with great friends Shaun Gillies and Tim Orchard.

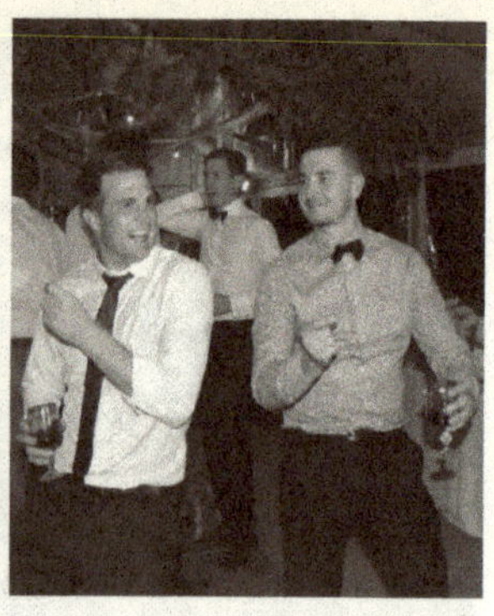

Having some fun with best mate Ben Fagan at a friend's wedding in 2015.

Duck has a younger brother, Matt. Matt and Tig were great mates and it was awesome to watch their friendship blossom over the years. Since losing Ty I've watched how close Matt and Duck have become. I'm sure some of it has to do with watching me go through the loss of Ty. I've left their house after watching them laugh, care, and be kind to each other. When I see them like that I can't help but get emotional and regret that I didn't get that opportunity with Ty. But as the years go on I see it as one of the many blessings and lessons Ty left for me.

I'm glad now I understand more about mental health and mental illness. I've been guilty of making jokes about depression, of saying the word like it means nothing. Before Ty died I would talk about wanting to kill myself because I had to work on a weekend. Or point a gun-finger at my temple as a joke. I never thought about the actual pain some people might be going through. I cringe now when I hear or see someone say or do that. People make these jokes and take it so lightly, when there are many people out there genuinely hating life, genuinely considering that action.

We all need to be more aware, more sensitive and more supportive of those who are doing it tough. They'll never feel comfortable opening up and getting help if the community around them are joking about it, making fun of their feelings, or calling them 'crazy' or 'weak' or 'strange.'

WHEN I THINK long term about SPEAK UP! Stay ChatTY, I am 100 per cent clear where I want it to go: more programs, more staff, more community engagement, more ways we can open up the conversation about mental health and suicide.

But I'm not 100 per cent sure on how I want to be connected to the organisation in the future. I wonder if I can always make a career out of dwelling in the past. I don't know if I can fully move forward if I'm frozen in that moment of my life. I might start to burn out from sharing my story, and might eventually want to move on. For now, though, it is great. I love my team, I love my making a difference, and each day I go home with a real sense of achievement that I know I am lucky to have.

I still dream big about Stay ChatTY and will always work hard to grow it. But, as a realist, I know not all things pan out how you might want them to. Not-for-profit is a saturated market and flavours can change very quickly. Nevertheless, I hope that in years to come I am sitting on the board of this organisation helping to make decisions for the betterment of lives across Australia.

In August 2017 I toured nationally with the RUOK? "conversation convoy". RUOK? is a mental health movement in Australia, reminding people that meaningful conversations can save lives. Aussie ambassadors from the stage, screen and media hit the road for six weeks, travelling 14,000 km around the

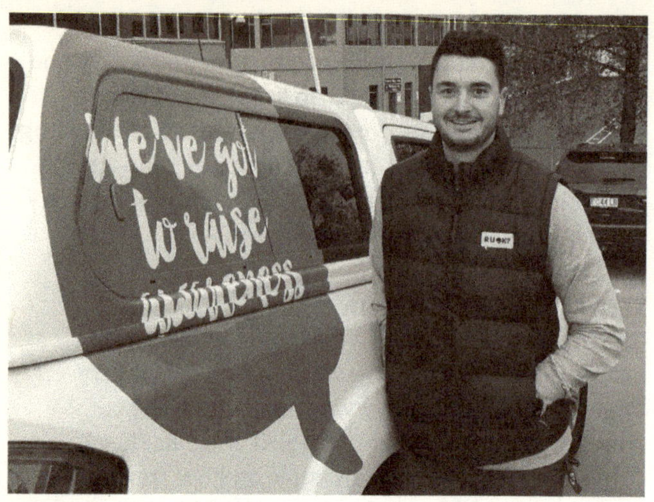

I am a proud ambassador for National Mental Health Organisation RUOK?. The friends and contacts I have made since becoming part of this amazing team is something that I truly value.

country to promote having healthy conversations and checking in with your friends. I was lucky enough to spend time with Australian actor and director Steve Bastoni, also an ambassador for RUOK?.

Many people would envy Steve's past. He used to party like mad, associate with Australia's biggest celebrity names and lived the absolute high life. But at one stage, his wife went through a tough time and needed him to be there for her. He realised things needed to change. He needed to know more about mental health and suicide before it took away someone he loved.

The RUOK? convoy of cars had docked in Devonport; it was the final leg of the tour. After travelling overnight by boat from Melbourne, I shared the four-hour drive back home to Hobart with Steve. I had never met Steve before, but we got on well and had a laugh.

It was on that drive Steve said something to me I will always remember. Now, I see it as a turning point that helped me achieve a different outlook after losing Ty.

"Losing your brother is and probably will be the most devastating thing you experience," he said. "It fucking sucks." (He swore a lot.) "But the gift your brother gave to you was a purpose in life. Not everyone finds their purpose. In a roundabout way you are one of the lucky ones who's found your calling."

"Yeah, absolutely, I agree", I replied, but it was a lazy response and I'm not sure I really felt Steve's words in my heart. After the tour was over and I'd had time to reflect on such an amazing experience, Steve's words really hit home. I was moved because it was the first time I genuinely realised that my life did have a purpose.

Unfortunately for me, the person I loved the most, my best friend, died before I could realise my purpose. And it took that loss for me to find that purpose. When I think back to my life when Ty was alive, I ask myself, why didn't I have the drive to succeed and be who I want to be? Why didn't I explore my passions and let them lead me to new opportunities? I hate that it took my brother's death to unearth this drive. But as Steve said, I am lucky I found it. I am grateful that Ty has brought me here. I'm convinced I can share what I've learned to help shape the lives of other young Mitch McPhersons, and really make a meaningful difference.

No matter what happens, Stay ChatTY and that pair of shorts will always be around in one way or another. The work we have done and the things we have achieved in the past years will always linger in people's hearts and minds. If the conversation about those shorts encourages someone to open up to a friend or a loved one, we will have done what we set out to do. And that is something I will always be proud of.

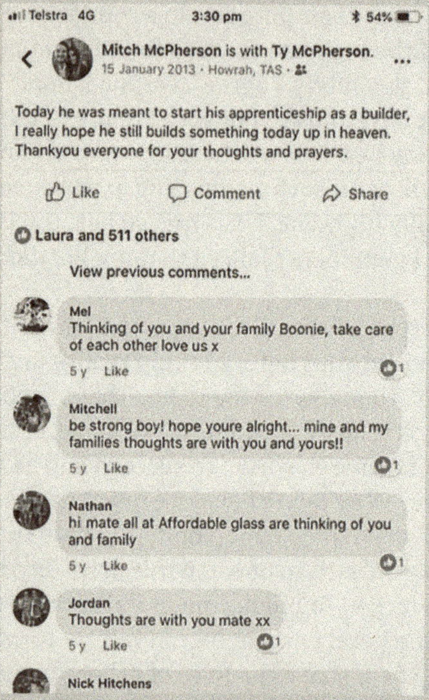

Telstra 4G 3:30 pm 54%

Mitch McPherson is with **Ty McPherson**.
15 January 2013 · Howrah, TAS

Today he was meant to start his apprenticeship as a builder, I really hope he still builds something today up in heaven. Thankyou everyone for your thoughts and prayers.

Like Comment Share

Laura and 511 others

View previous comments...

Mel
Thinking of you and your family Boonie, take care of each other love us x
5 y Like 1

Mitchell
be strong boy! hope youre alright... mine and my families thoughts are with you and yours!!
5 y Like 1

Nathan
hi mate all at Affordable glass are thinking of you and family
5 y Like 1

Jordan
Thoughts are with you mate xx
5 y Like 1

Nick Hitchens

The day after my little brother took his own life he was meant to start a building apprenticeship. This post shows the raw pain I felt in telling my Facebook friends of the tragic news.